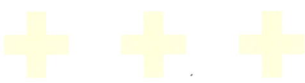

INTRODUCTION

If you've experienced anxiety at some point in your life, you're certainly not alone. Most people can recognize those uncomfortable telltale signs, such as worries spiralling in a loop around your head, "butterflies" in your stomach and a racing heart.

As uncomfortable as it can be, anxiety is actually a perfectly normal human emotion we all experience from time to time. After all, if you're about to sit an important exam, propose to your partner or bungee jump off a bridge, you're likely to feel a tad jittery (to say the least!). However, if your anxiety has become a daily occurrence, popping up in unnecessary situations and making peace of mind seem impossible... well, that's a different story altogether. It's also where this book comes in.

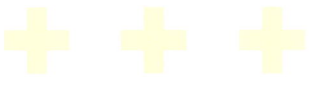

CONTENTS

Introduction	6
How to Use This Book	8
Chapter One: Anxiety 101	10
Chapter Two: Self and Health	46
Chapter Three: Social Situations	82
Chapter Four: The Wider World	118
Conclusion	152
Resources	154
Index	156

Disclaimer

Neither the author nor the publisher can be held responsible for any injury, loss or claim – be it health, financial or otherwise – arising out of the use, or misuse, of the suggestions made herein. This book is not intended as a substitute for the medical advice of a doctor or physician. If you are experiencing problems with your physical or mental health, it is always best to follow the advice of a medical professional.

ANXIETY
FIRST-AID KIT

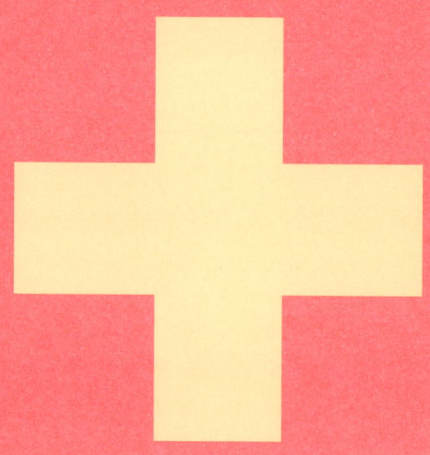

Tips and Techniques to Help You
Manage Anxiety in Any Situation

CLAIRE CHAMBERLAIN

ANXIETY FIRST-AID KIT

Copyright © Octopus Publishing Group Limited, 2026

All rights reserved.

No part of this book may be reproduced by any means, nor transmitted, nor translated into a machine language, without the written permission of the publishers.

Claire Chamberlain has asserted their right to be identified as the author of this work in accordance with sections 77 and 78 of the Copyright, Designs and Patents Act 1988.

Condition of Sale
This book is sold subject to the condition that it shall not, by way of trade or otherwise, be lent, resold, hired out or otherwise circulated in any form of binding or cover other than that in which it is published and without a similar condition including this condition being imposed on the subsequent purchaser.

An Hachette UK Company
www.hachette.co.uk

Vie Books, an imprint of Summersdale Publishers
Part of Octopus Publishing Group Limited
Carmelite House
50 Victoria Embankment
LONDON
EC4Y 0DZ
UK

This FSC® label means that materials and other controlled sources used for the product have been responsibly sourced

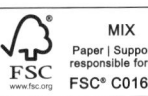

www.summersdale.com

The authorized representative in the EEA is Hachette Ireland, 8 Castlecourt Centre, Dublin 15, D15 XTP3, Ireland (email: info@hbgi.ie)

Printed and bound in China

ISBN: 978-1-83799-753-4
eISBN: 978-1-83799-754-1

Substantial discounts on bulk quantities of Summersdale books are available to corporations, professional associations and other organizations. For details contact general enquiries: telephone: +44 (0) 1243 771107 or email: enquiries@summersdale.com.

ANXIETY FIRST-AID KIT

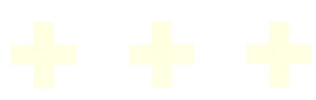

The *Anxiety First-Aid Kit* is designed to help you understand the root cause of your anxiety and offers a series of practical tips, inspiring ideas and step-by-step exercises, all with the aim of helping you manage and regain control over your anxiety before it becomes more serious. Covering a wide range of anxiety-inducing scenarios, from worries about health and body image, to social scenarios such as meeting new people and making phone calls, right through to political, financial and eco-anxiety, the advice in these pages aims to help you understand why it's happening, while the tips and techniques offer you quick, practical remedies for when you need some on-the-spot anxiety first aid.

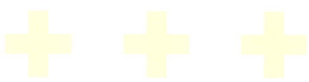

HOW TO USE THIS BOOK

As we've mentioned, anxiety can be a normal – even healthy – part of life, helping to keep you safe and steer you away from potentially dangerous situations. If, however, your anxiety has become all-consuming, or if it's started interfering with the way you'd like to live your life, then the *Anxiety First-Aid Kit* is for you! Inside, you'll find:

+ Information on anxiety disorders, symptoms and triggers.
+ Simple and easy-to-implement coping strategies for a wide range of anxiety-inducing situations.
+ Guided meditations and breathing exercises to help induce a sense of ease and calm.

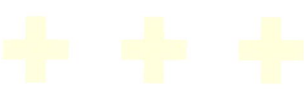

The information in Chapter One is designed to give you a broad understanding of what anxiety is and why it's affecting you, while the subsequent chapters are divided into three categories: self and health, social situations and the wider world. There's no right or wrong way to dive into this book – read it from cover to cover, or use the handy index to search for the issues most relevant to you, and then home in on the tips and exercises that are tailored to your needs.

However you approach it, the *Anxiety First-Aid Kit* is here to offer you comfort and relief from those niggling (and sometimes debilitating) anxiety symptoms. Are you ready? Then let the healing begin...

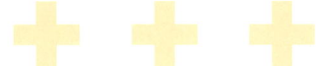

CHAPTER ONE:

ANXIETY 101

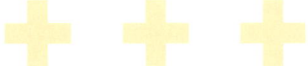

Have you ever been in a situation – perhaps before stepping into an exam hall or after reading a newspaper article – and begun to feel a sense of discomfort or panic? Discomfort or panic that made your heart race, your palms sweat and your stomach feel nauseous? This is anxiety and, while there isn't a one-size-fits-all experience, it does tend to present with a fairly typical set of symptoms.

In this chapter, we'll explore these often uncomfortable physical and emotional symptoms in more depth, as well as the reasons they might occur and some common anxiety disorders. You'll also find some quick and effective go-to fixes for when your anxiety begins to spiral – think of it as instant anxiety first aid for when you need it most.

WHAT IS ANXIETY?

Anxiety is not a rigid black-or-white experience. Instead, it exists on a sliding scale of grey. It tends to be characterized by feelings of unease or worry, often in relation to future or imagined events, and can be mild, moderate or – in some cases – severe and debilitating.

It's important to remember that anxiety can be a normal response to certain stressful situations (such as walking into a job interview). Most people also experience anxiety during periods of change or uncertainty. However, if you've started feeling anxious on a daily basis, your anxiety seems out of proportion to the situations you're facing, or if it's started affecting your sleep or the way you'd like to live your life (for example, you avoid certain places, events or social gatherings because of your anxiety), it might be time to take proactive steps to start feeling better.

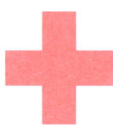

COMMON SYMPTOMS OF ANXIETY

Anxiety comes with a range of symptoms, both mental and physical. These include (but are not limited to):

+ A racing heart.
+ "Butterflies" in your stomach.
+ Nausea.
+ Dizziness.
+ Quick, shallow breathing.
+ Excessive worrying.
+ Feelings of dissociation.
+ Panic attacks.
+ Agitation.

The intensity of these symptoms can vary wildly. Acute and severe physical symptoms, such as a racing heart and even chest pain, can sometimes make you feel like you're experiencing a serious health issue, such as a heart attack. Understanding what is happening and how to get your symptoms under control with easy and effective calming measures can be crucial to your well-being.

ANXIETY VERSUS WORRY

Do you ever wonder whether you really have anxiety, or whether it's just good old everyday worry? Because everyone worries, right?

While the two are closely linked – excessive worrying can certainly be a common anxiety symptom – there is a difference.

Worrying is a temporary state of overthinking that everyone suffers from occasionally. It's usually attached to a specific upcoming event, such as making a wedding speech or delivering a work presentation, or being stuck between choices, such as which universities to apply for. Worry tends to be fairly temporary, passing once the event has happened or the decision has been made.

If you're struggling with anxiety, however, it will arise regardless of your current or upcoming circumstances and, while it will cause you to worry (perhaps uncontrollably), you'll also experience other symptoms, such as those listed on page 13, including nausea, dizziness or a racing pulse.

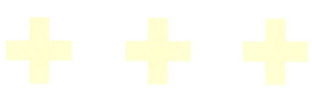

ANXIETY'S ORIGINS

If anxiety is so uncomfortable, why do we get caught up in it? From an evolutionary perspective, anxiety is the body's alert system, warning us about potential threats. A precursor to the fight, flight or freeze response, anxiety is a warning that something important warrants our attention. Historically, anxiety alerted us to life-threatening situations, such as running out of food or an imminent predator attack.

While modern-day anxiety can be helpful – for example, by motivating us to study for an exam – it can feel extreme. That's because, while the anxiety response is real, modern-day triggers have changed. These days, we're not about to be attacked by a sabre-toothed tiger, but simply trying to find a parking space or the courage to make a phone call. This is why a little anxiety first aid is useful, to help manage those symptoms that are out of proportion with our reality.

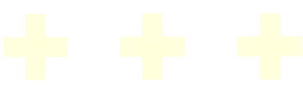

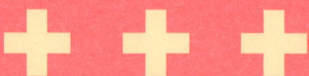

COMMON ANXIETY TRIGGERS

There are many triggers that cause anxiety, both internal and external, and yours will be unique to you. Even if you feel like anxiety catches you off guard, popping up from nowhere, a little digging beneath the surface often reveals a link to something more deep-seated and internalized.

For example, if your anxiety kicks in when you're asked to give a short presentation at work, you might feel it stems from worrying about messing up in front of your colleagues. Dig a little deeper, and you might find this matters to you because you hold the belief that you must be perfect all the time, which might be rooted in low self-worth, making you feel like you're not good enough. Or perhaps a childhood experience, such as falling over on stage during a school production, has instilled a fear of being in the spotlight.

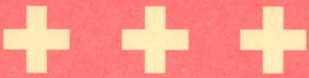

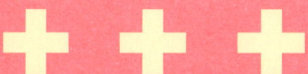

A huge array of external triggers can lead to anxiety spiralling out of control. Along with having to give a presentation at college or work, common triggers include:

+ Talking on the phone.
+ Flying in a plane.
+ Going to the doctor or dentist.
+ Having to make small talk at a party.
+ Driving somewhere new.
+ Moving house.
+ Lack of sleep.
+ Political uncertainty.
+ Climate change.

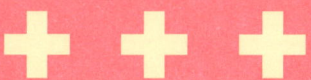

WHO GETS ANXIETY?

While most people experience anxious thoughts now and then, chronic anxiety is a mental health condition that can heavily impact your life. The World Health Organization reports that anxiety disorders are the most common mental health disorders worldwide, affecting 301 million people globally. And even if you haven't been diagnosed with a disorder, your experience of anxiety is completely valid. All of which means that anxiety is common and you're not alone. However, this absolutely does not mean you have to simply accept it and get on with life as best you can, despite the uncomfortable (and sometimes debilitating) symptoms. Far from it! As you'll see later in this book, a little anxiety first aid can go a LONG way! But before we dive into some helpful remedies, first we'll look at some common anxiety disorders, to help you get a handle on what's really going on…

ANXIETY DISORDERS

Anxiety disorders are a group of mental health conditions that cause feelings of extreme fear, dread and other symptoms that we explored on page 13, which are out of proportion to the situation. Depending on the types of symptoms you're currently experiencing, or have experienced in the past, it's possible you have a specific anxiety disorder.

Some of the most common anxiety disorders diagnosed by medical professionals include generalized anxiety disorder, social anxiety disorder, panic disorder, illness anxiety disorder, phobias, obsessive compulsive disorder and post-traumatic stress disorder. We'll explore these in more detail over the following pages and, if you read something that sounds familiar, try not to worry – anxiety disorders usually respond well to treatment, so don't be afraid to reach out to your health professional.

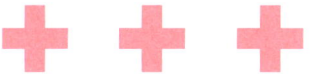

GENERALIZED ANXIETY DISORDER

If you experience chronic anxiety relating to a wide range of situations and events, you may be suffering with generalized anxiety disorder (GAD). As the name suggests, this disorder is general and all-encompassing and can lead you to feel anxious most of the time. Your worries might seem uncontrollable and can bring on symptoms such as restlessness, unease, irritability, dread and trouble sleeping.

While GAD can make you feel like you're the odd one out and that no one else could possibly be experiencing such extreme and constant anxiety, you're not the only one going through it: the NHS estimates 5 per cent of the UK population suffer with GAD, while in the US, data from National Comorbidity Survey Replication suggests 5.7 per cent of American adults experience it at some point in their lives.

SOCIAL ANXIETY DISORDER

More than simply feeling shy, social anxiety disorder is characterized by an overwhelming fear of social situations, which can negatively impact your life. Common symptoms include worrying excessively about everyday activities, such as meeting new people, going to work or the shops, or speaking on the phone; anxiety about going to restaurants and eating in public; fear of social situations, including times you might have to mingle or make small talk; and worries about being noticed. Physical symptoms can include blushing, nausea and panic attacks (see page 24). Because it involves fear of going out, social anxiety disorder can lead to loneliness, isolation and low self-esteem if you start withdrawing from situations that cause you fear.

If you struggle with social anxiety disorder, we have lots of tips to help with specific situations, such as talking on the phone, in Chapter Three, from page 82.

ILLNESS ANXIETY DISORDER

Also known as health anxiety, illness anxiety disorder is characterized by worrying that you're ill – or about to get ill – so much so that it takes over your life. Related to obsessive compulsive disorder (see page 25), symptoms include:

+ Constantly worrying that you're ill and checking your body for signs of illness.
+ Frequently searching for symptoms and their causes online.
+ Making frequent medical appointments.
+ Not feeling reassured by appointments or negative test results.
+ Avoiding people, places or activities for fear of contracting an illness.

Physical symptoms of anxiety, such as headaches, can exacerbate these symptoms. If you feel like you might have illness anxiety disorder, talking therapy can help to determine its origin. Also helpful are the ideas at the end of this chapter, such as deep breathing (page 36) and mindfulness (page 38).

The weirdest thing about a mind is that you can have the most intense things going on in there, but no one else can see them.

MATT HAIG

PANIC ATTACKS (AND PANIC DISORDER)

If you've ever had a panic attack, you'll know how distressing they can be. They're characterized by an abrupt onset of intense fear that usually lasts between 5 and 20 minutes. Symptoms often build quickly and include a racing heart, shallow breathing, trembling, sweating, chest pain and the sense you might collapse. If you have recurrent, unexpected panic attacks, you might be experiencing panic disorder.

The following anxiety first aid can help in the middle of an attack:

+ Focus on breathing slowly and deeply.
+ Stamp on the spot.
+ Focus on each of your senses in turn.
+ Carry a small comforting object with you, such as a worry stone or cuddly toy.
+ Try a grounding technique, such as the 3-3-3 technique on page 44.

OBSESSIVE COMPULSIVE DISORDER

If your anxiety presents as cycles of recurring and obsessive thoughts that lead to repetitive compulsions, you may be suffering with obsessive compulsive disorder (OCD). With OCD, the drive to perform compulsive behaviours is strong. Compulsions will be unique to you, but common ones include hand washing, checking doors are locked, counting and repeating words in your head. While compulsions might temporarily ease feelings of stress, ultimately these ritualistic behaviours can take over your life, interfering with daily activities and causing significant anxiety. Breaking the cycle can seem scary, but help is available, usually in the form of talking therapy and medication. OCD first-aid can include distraction techniques, such as doing something creative, watching a film, focusing on each of your senses or the 3-3-3 technique (page 44), or visualization techniques (page 42).

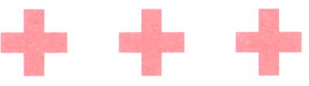

POST-TRAUMATIC STRESS DISORDER

Many people who experience or witness a traumatic event will need time to come to terms with it. But if you experience intrusive memories (such as flashbacks), negative mood swings, or changes in physical or emotional reactions (such as insomnia or irritability), and these symptoms last for a while and/or worsen over time, you may be experiencing post-traumatic stress disorder (PTSD). This form of anxiety can be triggered by sudden reminders, such as the sound of fireworks. Treatment is important and can include psychotherapy, exposure therapy, cognitive restructuring and/or medication. There are some first-aid steps you can take to help yourself, though: tell a friend or relative what you're going through, avoid alcohol, maintain a regular sleep routine, practise mindfulness (page 38), exercise regularly and be gentle with yourself – PTSD will likely ease gradually, not instantly.

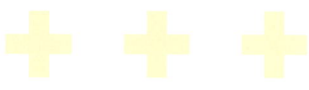

COMPARISON SYNDROME

If you frequently worry that others are having rewarding, fulfilling experiences while you're not, you may be suffering from comparison syndrome. The anxiety caused by comparison syndrome is very real, as you constantly compare yourself to your peers – often unfavourably. You might start to believe you're not as successful, attractive or adventurous as others.

Comparison syndrome often strongly correlates with high social media usage. If you feel like the anxiety related to comparison syndrome is damaging your mental health, try these first-aid tips:

+ Schedule in some social-media-free time each day – even just half an hour.
+ Instead of scrolling, try reading, drawing, going for a walk or yoga.
+ Remember, no one's real life looks the way it does on social media.
+ Talk to someone you trust about how social media is making you feel.

PHOBIAS

A phobia is an anxiety disorder characterized by feelings of intense fear in relation to a particular place, object, situation or animal. To be classed as a phobia, the fear must be overwhelming, out of proportion and persistent, lasting for six months or more. Alongside feelings of fear, symptoms of phobias include a racing heart, shortened breath, dizziness, sweating, trembling and nausea. The symptoms will only arise when you experience the subject of your phobia. The rest of the time, you'll likely be able to get on with your life without disruption.

Phobias can be split into two main categories: specific (simple) phobias and complex phobias.

Specific (simple) phobias

These phobias centre around a particular trigger, which can be an animal (such as dogs or spiders), environmental (such as heights), situational (such as flying), bodily (such as vomit) or sexual (such as performance anxiety). These types of phobias often develop during adolescence and may lessen as you get older.

Complex phobias

These phobias tend to be deep-rooted and develop during adulthood. The main complex phobias are agoraphobia (fear of being out and about, including in large crowds) and social phobia (also known as social anxiety disorder, which we've looked at on page 21).

Anxiety first aid for phobias

Specific treatments may be required to help you rid yourself of your phobia for good, such as medications, talking therapies and/or exposure therapy. It is important to speak to your doctor if a phobia is impacting your life in a big way. There are also some self-help remedies you can try: relaxation techniques, such as breathing exercises (page 36), meditation (page 40) and visualizations (page 42) can all help you practise staying calm, so that when you're faced with your phobia, it doesn't impact you so severely.

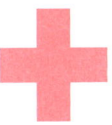

THE STRESS OF MODERN LIVING

It is not only people with a diagnosed disorder who experience anxiety. The pace of life has accelerated so rapidly in recent times that many of us experience stress and anxiety in relation to modernity on a daily basis. No longer led by our natural rhythms and body clock, we tend to work longer hours, expose ourselves to increased screen time, move less and spend fewer hours outside in the natural world, which can all take its toll on both our minds and bodies. Learning to slow down or pause, even for a moment, can help to counteract this frenetic pace of life. From page 32, you'll find some first-aid ideas on how to slow down and lower your stress levels to help reduce or alleviate everyday anxiety.

THE PRESSURE TO BE "PERFECT"

The pressure to be all things to all people can be a source of anxiety for many. Expectations (that we often place on ourselves) to be the perfect parent, employee, partner or friend can leave us feeling stretched too thin. Of course, having a fulfilling career and great social life is brilliant, but if we're chasing these things to the detriment of our own health, it can leave us feeling anxious. Here are a few first-aid tips to help you wean yourself off trying to be perfect so you can restore some mental balance:

+ Delegate work projects if possible.
+ Enlist support from a partner or family member at home.
+ Practise saying "no" (more about this on page 114).
+ Don't feel guilty for prioritizing yourself sometimes.

CALMING COPING STRATEGIES

Hopefully by this point, you'll have realized that when it comes to anxiety, you're not alone. And even if your anxiety is severe or you've been diagnosed with a specific anxiety disorder, there are professional treatments available to help you overcome it (see page 45). Keeping in mind that anxiety is both treatable and manageable can provide reassurance and stave off fears that you'll have to suffer with it forever.

Self-care techniques are hugely important for the management of anxiety, acting as anxiety first aid for in-the-moment relief when you're struggling. Over the following pages, we'll explore some strategies you can turn to whenever anxiety takes hold.

A LITTLE SELF-CARE CAN CREATE THE CALM YOU DESIRE

TRY REFRAMING YOUR ANXIETY

It might sound strange at first, but reframing your anxiety as something helpful and positive can be a powerful first-aid strategy. Because however uncomfortable, annoying, frustrating or even debilitating your anxiety might be at times, it's actually trying to be useful. Sounds odd, right? But let's think back to the origins of anxiety, which we looked at on page 15. Feelings of anxiety evolved in our ancestors when they needed to stay safe. For example, seeing a predator would make them feel anxious, instigating the fight, flight or freeze response necessary to help them act appropriately and, therefore, stay alive. Your own anxiety is trying to do this for you, to help you stay safe.

For instance, think about a time when you tend to feel anxious – perhaps before catching up with a group of friends you haven't seen in a while. Those symptoms of anxiety – including a racing heart and shallow breathing – might be horrible, but ultimately the worry you experience before meeting up is likely to inspire you to brush up on your small talk to give you the confidence to join the conversation. And the nerves you feel? That's partly down to your body releasing a surge of adrenaline to heighten your alertness and give you the energy you need to enjoy yourself.

Remembering why your mind and body are making you anxious – and even feeling grateful for the experience – can help you come to terms with anxiety and to thrive whenever anxiety rears its head. Getting into the routine of reminding yourself why you feel anxious – and often it's only because you care about something – is a go-to first-aid tip that can really help.

BREATHE DEEPLY

Gently slowing and lengthening your breath is a centuries-old practice to help calm the mind and body and lessen feelings of anxiety. It's one of the simplest forms of self-care, and it is something you can do anywhere. Breathing deeply works by triggering your parasympathetic nervous system (which is responsible for feelings of relaxation) and interrupting the sympathetic nervous system (which creates all those fight, flight or freeze responses). Mindful deep breathing is simple to perform – follow these steps whenever you feel your anxiety beginning to spiral:

1. Begin by tuning into your breathing.
2. Start to consciously slow and lengthen each breath. Inhale for 5 seconds, hold for 1 second, exhale for 5 seconds, hold for a final second.
3. Repeat for ten breaths, or longer if needed.

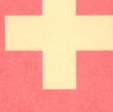

REPEAT A MANTRA

A mantra is a simple saying or slogan you can repeat whenever you feel you need a reminder to stay calm, clear-headed and present. Repeating daily mantras has been shown to help rewire your thoughts and create positive feelings or intentions, and this anxiety first-aid strategy can be used to interrupt a cycle of fear-based negative thoughts. Effective mantras to help combat anxiety should be short, simple and easy to remember. You could try some of the following – simply repeat slowly to yourself, in your head or out loud (in an appropriate environment), until you feel your mind begin to calm:

+ "This too shall pass."
+ "I've got this."
+ "I deserve peace and happiness."
+ "I can do difficult things."
+ "I am enough exactly as I am."

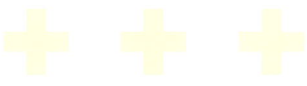

STAY IN THE PRESENT MOMENT

Have you ever noticed that when you're feeling anxious your mind usually races ahead of you, worrying about a future event that may or may not happen? Or perhaps your mind is going over and over a past event, listing the numerous ways you could have done something differently. This tends to be the nature of anxiety – it centres around fears of future scenarios or worries about things that have already happened. This is why it can feel so free-floating and hard to control: because you can't do anything practical to resolve a problem that hasn't happened yet (if it does at all) or go back and change the past.

Grounding yourself in the present moment (in other words, practising mindfulness) can really help to ease anxiety. Giving your full attention to "right now" means there's no room to ruminate on the past or worry about the future. The more you place the focus of your attention on the present moment, the more you'll find anxiety cannot exist in the same space as conscious awareness.

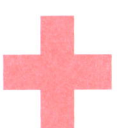

To start drawing your attention back to the present moment in times of anxiety, try the following:

+ Focus fully on the rhythm of your breathing. You could try slowing and lengthening each breath (see page 36).

+ If you're sitting, standing or walking, focus on the feeling of your feet pressing down on the ground.

+ Really pay attention to your surroundings: what small details can you notice that perhaps you haven't seen before?

+ Tune in to each of your senses in turn: what can you see, hear, smell, feel and even taste?

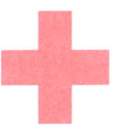

TRY MEDITATION

If you struggle with anxiety, you will likely benefit from building a meditation practice into your daily life. It doesn't have to take lots of time, either – spending just 5 or 10 minutes each day sitting quietly in meditation can do wonders for your well-being. In fact, according to research, a regular meditation practice can result in reduced stress and enhanced self-awareness, leaving you in a better place to manage everything life throws at you.

At its core, meditation is simply focused attention. There are many different ways to meditate, but one of the most common is to focus on your breath. Follow this easy step-by-step guide to complete your first meditation session:

1. Ensure you're in a quiet place, then sit comfortably, either on a chair with your feet flat on the floor or cross-legged on the floor.

2. Gently close your eyes.

3. Inhale deeply through your nose, then exhale fully, relaxing your shoulders down as you do so.

4. Now breathe normally, paying attention to each inhale and exhale. Don't try to change your breathing pattern or force yourself to breathe more deeply than normal.

5. If you find your mind wanders away from your breath, don't worry – this is normal. As soon as you notice your attention has shifted, simply draw your attention back to your breath.

6. If you struggle to focus on the breath, you could try counting each breath as follows: inhale one, exhale two, inhale three, exhale four. Do this up to a count of ten, then return to one and repeat.

7. Pay attention to your breath for 5–10 minutes.

8. To finish, take one final deep inhale through your nose, then exhale through your mouth.

9. Slowly open your eyes.

ESCAPE THROUGH VISUALIZATION

Visualization is a technique that harnesses the power of your imagination to induce a feeling of calm, which can help to ease anxiety. It involves using mental imagery to alter your thoughts, feeling and mood – a little like daydreaming, only with a more conscious train of thought.

As with meditation, there are different ways you can use visualization. You might visualize achieving a goal to help with motivation, for example. When seeking to ease feelings of anxiety, the guided imagery that helps should foster a sense of peace. The following step-by-step instructions will guide you through a simple visualization.

1. Ensure you're in a quiet place, then lie or sit comfortably.

2. Close your eyes.

3. Inhale deeply through your nose, then exhale fully.

4. Now, imagine you're lying on a beautiful beach*: the turquoise water is gently lapping

against the shore and the sand is warm beneath your body.

5. Feel the weight of your body relax as it rests upon the sand.
6. Listen to the sound of the waves, knowing you're completely safe and supported.
7. Feel your worries melt away as you lie on the beach and gently release any tension you might be holding in your body. Allow everything to soften and rest.
8. Slow your breathing, matching the rhythm of the waves.
9. Spend as much time here as you need, relaxing effortlessly.
10. When you're ready, imagine standing up and walking slowly away from the beach, knowing you can return to it at any time.
11. Slowly open your eyes.

*If a beach doesn't work for you, imagine a different space instead: a beautiful meadow, perhaps. Wherever you decide, be sure to visualize it fully: the sights, sounds and smells.

GROUND YOURSELF WITH THE 3-3-3 TECHNIQUE

Anxiety can leave you caught up in a whirlwind of panicked thoughts. The 3-3-3 technique shifts your attention back to your physical body in the present moment, leading to a calmer state of mind in minutes.

If you're experiencing a moment of acute anxiety, this quick but effective bit of first aid can help you to feel more grounded.

1. Take three deep breaths, inhaling slowly through your nose, then exhaling gently through your mouth.

2. Now, look around you and name three things you can see.

3. Next, name three things you can hear.

4. Finally, move three parts of your body. It could simply be gently rolling your shoulders a few times, clenching and unclenching your hands, then wiggling your toes. As you perform each movement, focus on the bodily sensations.

5. To finish, take three more deep breaths.

WHEN TO SEEK PROFESSIONAL SUPPORT

While the self-care ideas we've just explored – as well as those still to come – will hopefully help to ease your anxiety, this book is not a stand-in for expert medical advice. If you continue to struggle with anxiety, it's important to speak with your doctor, who will be able to offer support or diagnose an anxiety disorder. Make an appointment if:

+ Your anxiety is affecting your daily life or causing you distress.
+ Your worrying has become uncontrollable.
+ You regularly feel restless or on edge.
+ You have difficulty concentrating.
+ Your anxiety is causing sleep problems.

To prepare for your appointment, write down everything you want to discuss so you don't forget any crucial information. Your doctor may be able to discuss various treatments with you, such as talking therapy or medication.

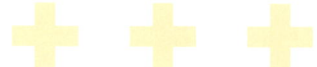

CHAPTER TWO:

SELF AND HEALTH

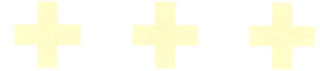

Anxiety can manifest in myriad ways related to the themes of self and health. From concerns around health and self-care issues – such as alcohol use, body image, appearance, ageing, sleep and periods – to worries about specific scenarios, such as going to the doctor or having your photo taken, there are so many situations that can cause us stress and anxiety.

This chapter will delve into some common anxieties around the themes of self and health. You will also find insights to help you understand your experiences, along with tips, techniques and step-by-step exercises to help you overcome your fears, worries and anxieties. With understanding comes the ability to move beyond the things that have been holding you back. It's time to reclaim your power!

ANXIETY AND BODY IMAGE

The relationship between anxiety and body image issues is complex. Just as having poor body image can increase feelings of anxiety and low self-worth, so too can anxiety increase the likelihood of poor body image. Everybody has a unique relationship with their body and how they view themselves, and as such, body image issues can be numerous and varied. For example, one person might feel anxious about something that marks them out as different, such as a birthmark, while someone else might have a dislike for a certain part of their body, and another may hate their body size or shape. Having anxiety alongside poor body image can, in some cases, lead to damaging decisions or behaviours. Over the following pages, we'll take a deeper dive into anxiety and body image to explore problems that can arise and how to work to overcome them.

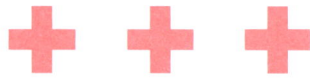

THE IMPACT OF ANXIETY AND POOR BODY IMAGE

Sadly, poor body image is becoming increasingly common in our image-obsessed world. Online, you might encounter a barrage of "perfect" celebrities and influencers on a daily basis, which can make you feel like you need to compete with or live up to their filtered, highly stylized images. If you have high self-esteem and good body image, along with a support network of family and friends who also model this mindset to you, it's unlikely these online encounters will bother you. But if you struggle with poor body image or you don't have a strong support network around you, the impact of media consumption and other societal pressures can manifest in negative, unhelpful and harmful ways. These can include disordered eating, an eating disorder or body dysmorphic disorder.

BODY DYSMORPHIC DISORDER

Body dysmorphic disorder (BDD) is sometimes dismissed as "vanity", but it is a serious and distressing anxiety-based mental health condition. Symptoms include comparing your appearance with other people's, disliking specific areas of your body, anxiety about your "flaws" (which are often imagined or imperceptible), spending considerable time trying to hide these "flaws" with make-up or clothes, obsessing with the idea of surgery and constantly checking mirrors or avoiding them altogether.

BDD can affect all genders. It's important to seek help if you recognize these symptoms in yourself; left unchecked, BDD can lead to social anxiety, depression, eating disorders, self-harm or even suicidal thoughts. Accessing therapy via your doctor or finding a local support group are important steps, but there are some anxiety first-aid techniques that can help too, including mindfulness (page 38), the 3-3-3 technique (page 44) and specific body image tips and affirmations (pages 52–53).

DISORDERED EATING AND EATING DISORDERS

Disordered eating and eating disorders are complex mental illnesses that often have strong links with anxiety. This is because anxiety disorders, such as social anxiety, OCD and GAD, can make a person feel as though they have no control – something they feel they can regain through restricted eating habits and excessive dieting. There are many contributing factors when a person struggles with disordered eating and eating disorders. The desire to be thin isn't always the cause, but poor body image and low self-esteem often play a part. While some of the anxiety first aid in this book might provide in-the-moment help with these problems (see pages 52–53), seeking professional help is vital when addressing the complex issues of disordered eating and eating disorders. You can find information about eating disorder support in the Resources section of this book.

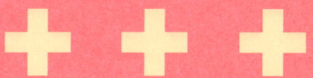

ANXIETY FIRST AID FOR BODY IMAGE

Poor body image can easily morph into something more sinister. If you recognize signs of BDD or disordered eating, or you're struggling to cope with poor body image on your own, it's important to gain professional support from your doctor, who will be able to offer confidential advice and possibly refer you for specialist help.

There are also steps you can take to help improve your body image so you can begin to embrace your fabulous uniqueness.

+ Talk kindly to yourself: sometimes, we are our own worst bullies. Every time you catch yourself speaking unkindly to yourself – perhaps telling yourself you're fat or ugly – stop immediately! Instead, remind yourself you're beautiful, unique and lovable.

+ Stop comparing yourself with others: from celebrities and models to influencers, we're all guilty of comparing ourselves with others now and then. But remind yourself, we don't all look like models – and we're not meant to! Each of us is unique, including you. Just imagine how boring life would be if we were all homogenized copies of each other. It's time to celebrate your individuality!

- + Switch your focus: instead of concentrating on how your body looks, focus on what it can do. After all, your body isn't here to be objectified, it's here to be moved and used! So go on that hike or swim in the sea if you're able to, savour some delicious food and hug someone you love. In short, throw yourself into the art of living.

- + Tell someone how you're feeling: if you're struggling, let someone close to you know how you've been feeling. Who can you open up to? Often, sharing your feelings is the first step to recovery.

FEAR OF HAVING YOUR PHOTO TAKEN

Being camera shy (scopophobia) can stem from not wanting to be seen, in some cases because of poor body image or not wishing to look "foolish". Being filmed rather than photographed can be even more difficult for those who are camera shy. Stepping before a lens requires vulnerability, which many find uncomfortable – we're not sure how we're going to be portrayed, so we become anxious about putting ourselves out there.

Like many phobias, camera shyness may have little impact on your life most of the time. But when a photograph of you is required, the fear can get real! If you suspect your camera shyness stems from struggles with body image, check out the tips on pages 52–53. Otherwise, these first-aid tips to overcome camera anxiety might help:

- Find a photographer you have a rapport with and explain your anxiety to them. If they're good at their job, they'll help put you at ease.

- Practice makes progress. Ask a trusted friend to take some snaps of you. Explain your worries so they understand, then arrange a quiet half hour together where you can get comfortable in front of the camera.

- Pull faces! If you're scared of looking "foolish", it's time to move past this by deliberately looking silly. Looking a bit daft on purpose can help you laugh and loosen up, so you appear more natural in your "for real" photos.

- Experiment with poses and angles. Try some head-on shots, as well as sitting at a 45-degree angle. Try some sitting shots and some standing, or have a friend stand behind the photographer so you can smile at them – it can make all the difference.

ANXIETY AND AGEING

From changes in metabolism and perimenopause, to hair loss, wrinkles and eyesight changes, small reminders that we're getting older will happen to all of us. Fear of ageing can sometimes be linked to body image issues, as our bodies change in ways we can't control. Our fears may be compounded by existential worries relating to purposelessness, frailty and mortality. All of this is often linked to fear of the unknown, as none of us knows what the future has in store.

Extreme fear of ageing (gerascophobia) can lead to irrational and obsessive thoughts, behaviours and compulsions, such as becoming fixated on health and fitness. Help can be found by learning how to cope with change and uncertainty, focusing on gratitude and using these anxiety first-aid tips:

+ Pay attention to right now, instead of some unknown point in the future. By embracing mindfulness (page 38), you can start appreciating all that's good in your life.

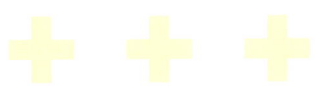

+ Accept the things you can't change. Yes, you're getting older, but we all are (if we're lucky). This is a fact of life, so aim to enjoy each day and everything you're able to do.

+ Start viewing ageing as a privilege. Many people aren't lucky enough to live to a ripe old age. Taking time to feel grateful for each day can make a difference.

+ Switch your mindset. Often when people think of getting older, they focus on the negatives and the things they might lose. Instead, think of everything you have to gain as you age, as well as all the experiences ahead of you. Remember, life doesn't stop at 50, 60, 70 or beyond, nor does it stop when you retire or when your children leave home. Start planning all the adventures you can still have!

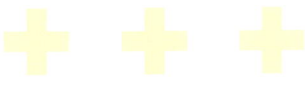

ANXIETY AND ALCOHOL OR DRUG USE

Anxiety and alcohol or drug use can become intricately linked in a complex cycle. Perhaps you turn to alcohol or drugs to "take the edge off" your anxiety. Is regular drinking or drug use giving you "hangxiety"? It could be a bit of both.

Be honest: have you ever tried to lessen your anxiety by pouring yourself an alcoholic drink to "unwind"? The trouble is, this type of "unwinding" masks or numbs your anxiety, rather than dealing with it. While alcohol and some drugs can make you feel relaxed in the short term, research shows that they increase feelings of anxiety. Further problems occur when numbing becomes chronic – even compulsive – and it can lead to addiction. If you're concerned about your alcohol or drug use, it's important to contact your doctor for confidential support, before trying the first-aid tips over the page.

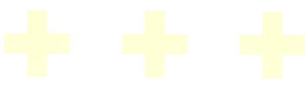

Living with anxiety – living alarmed – makes it impossible to enter the moment, to land inside my body and be there.

GLENNON DOYLE

ANXIETY FIRST AID FOR ALCOHOL AND DRUG USE

If alcohol or drugs are fuelling your anxiety, or if you've noticed you're indulging compulsively as a way of numbing your anxiety, now might be a good time to evaluate your relationship with them to develop healthier habits and coping mechanisms. Check out these alcohol and drug anxiety first-aid tips to get started:

+ Ask for help if you need to. If you're finding giving up alcohol or drugs more challenging than you thought you would, there's no shame in asking for help. Your doctor will be able to provide confidential advice and support, so make an appointment.

+ Decide you're going to drink or use drugs less often – or that you're going to give up altogether. Often, because of their addictive nature, it can be easier to steer clear entirely. Making a clear, conscious decision to change your habits is important because it acts as a promise to yourself. You could write down your decision to give up alcohol or drugs and stick it somewhere visible.

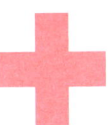

- Find your motivation – this is the reason you want to change your habits. Perhaps your anxiety has begun to spiral and you want to stop this, or you're realizing you're beginning to damage your health, finances and relationships. Maybe your motivation, then, is wanting to improve your health, sleep, bank balance and friendships. Keep these reasons in mind – they will keep you going.

- Don't berate yourself if you slip up. No one is perfect. If you do have a drink or take drugs while aiming not to, it's okay. It's not a reason to give up your resolution to change. This is an ongoing process, not an "all or nothing" thing.

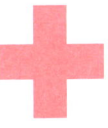

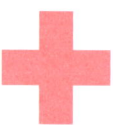

+ Get support from friends or family. Knowing people are on your side and will be there to support you will make it so much easier.

+ Take it one day at a time. As with many things in life, looking at the bigger picture or trying to project way into the future is only going to make you feel overwhelmed and even more anxious. Instead, simply focus on the here and now and the decisions you can make in this moment.

+ Celebrate each small win. Changing an ingrained habit is challenging, so celebrate each milestone, however small. You can also reward yourself with something that you love – a relaxing bubble bath, a new book or a meal out with a friend.

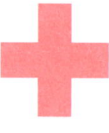

VISITING THE DOCTOR

Fear of visiting the doctor – also known as iatrophobia or "white coat syndrome" – is a common cause of anxiety. Research suggests that 15 to 30 per cent of people suffer from it. People cite many reasons for their fear, from anxiety about test results to feelings of powerlessness. There are some anxiety first-aid measures you can take, though, to help calm your mind when visiting the doctor.

+ Take a family member or friend to your appointment for support.

+ Do some breathing exercises in the waiting room (such as the exercise on page 36).

+ Repeat a positive mantra to yourself, such as: "Being here is the biggest form of self-care."

+ Tell your doctor you're nervous – they will want to help put you at ease. And remember, your doctor is just a regular person!

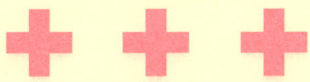

ANXIETY AND YOUR MENSTRUAL CYCLE

If you have a menstrual cycle, you might notice your anxiety fluctuates with your cycle. Because of fluctuating levels of oestrogen and progesterone during the luteal phase of your cycle (which usually begins around day 15 and ends when you get your period), you can feel low, anxious and sensitive around this time. Anxiety is also a common symptom of premenstrual syndrome (PMS) and can be severe. If it feels completely overwhelming, you might be experiencing premenstrual dysphoric disorder (PMDD), which is often described as severe PMS.

To identify whether your anxiety fluctuates with your cycle, it can be worth keeping a diary of when anxiety strikes and what seems to trigger it. This can help you spot a pattern, and is especially helpful if you experience free-floating anxiety (anxiety that you can't seem to pin to a certain event or experience).

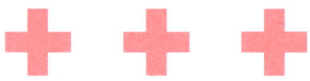

ANXIETY FIRST AID FOR PEOPLE WITH MENSTRUAL CYCLES

Anxiety related to your menstrual cycle can feel overwhelming but, as with other challenging aspects of your cycle, it's possible to manage your symptoms.

+ Keep a diary of your cycle and symptoms. This will help you spot the pattern, so you can start to predict when your anxiety will hit.

+ Be kind to yourself. Now you understand why you're feeling anxious, be gentle with yourself and remind yourself it will pass.

+ Take regular exercise throughout your cycle. This can help to manage and regulate PMS symptoms, including mood swings.

+ Opt for a healthy diet, including plenty of fresh vegetables and fruit.

+ If you smoke, now's the time to quit – smoking has been shown to worsen PMS symptoms.

+ Aim to get a good night's sleep each night. If you struggle, there's advice over the page.

ANXIETY AND SLEEP

Sleep is a vital physiological process that repairs your body and restores good mental function each night. But unfortunately, anxiety and a good night's sleep don't tend to go hand in hand. This is because your body's fight, flight or freeze mode – which you might have been in for most of the day due to an anxious, racing mind – isn't conducive to drifting off peacefully at night.

Poor sleep and sleep disturbances, including insomnia, regular night waking and the inability to fall into a deep sleep, have long been associated with feelings of anxiety and anxiety disorders. There are several reasons for this:

+ According to the Sleep Foundation, people with anxiety disorders are more likely to have higher sleep reactivity, which means they are much more prone to sleep problems when dealing with stress.

- Anxiety and sleep problems can create a vicious cycle: the more anxious you feel, the more you will struggle to sleep, but the less good-quality sleep you get, the worse your anxiety can become.
- The inability to get a good night's sleep can actually cause you to start dreading bedtime, which heightens your feelings of stress and anxiety, making it even harder to drift off.

While this vicious cycle can sound never-ending, it is possible to gently get your sleep back on track. Over the next few pages, we'll take a look at some tips and techniques that can help.

HOW TO CREATE A CALMING BEDTIME ROUTINE

If your anxiety is stopping you from sleeping, getting into good bedtime habits (also known as "sleep hygiene") can help. This is because your brain likes routine, and performing a set of bedtime rituals at roughly the same time each day sends a signal to your brain to start preparing for sleep. However, try not to get too hung up on the end result (namely, sleep). Putting pressure on yourself to nod off can increase your anxiety, which can undo your hard work. Instead, try adopting a relaxing, restful evening routine, placing emphasis on the pleasure of taking care of yourself. The following ideas can be a tonic for the sleep-deprived, providing sleep first aid to soothe the soul.

+ Avoid caffeine from midday.

+ Resist the temptation to stare at screens in the hour before bedtime, as the blue light they emit messes with your levels of sleep-inducing melatonin. Try setting a 60-minute device-free rule before bedtime.

- Dim the lights for half an hour before going to bed. Just as with the blue light from devices, bright lights can disrupt your melatonin levels.

- Aim to get to bed at roughly the same time each night.

- Be consistent with your routine. Follow the same steps in the same order each night, for example: putting your pyjamas on, reading your book for 20 minutes, brushing your teeth and performing a sleep meditation (see page 70) once you're under the covers.

- Try a warm, relaxing bath or shower before bed – the heat will help to relax your muscles, while the subsequent drop in body temperature when you get out can help to induce sleep.

- Make sure your bedroom is well ventilated by leaving a window partially open, as this can help you drift off.

YOUR STEP-BY-STEP SLEEP MEDITATION GUIDE

Evidence suggests that a regular sleep meditation practice may improve sleep quality, alongside good sleep hygiene habits and a bedtime routine. Try the following sleep meditation to help you drift off at night:

1. Lie down in bed beneath your covers, ensuring that you're comfortable. Make sure the lights are switched off.

2. Gently close your eyes.

3. Take three deep breaths, inhaling deeply through your nose and exhaling fully through your mouth.

4. Now, gently focus attention on your toes. Spend a few moments imagining the muscles in your toes relaxing fully after a busy day.

5. Next, gently move your attention to your feet. Feel them getting heavy as they relax fully.

6. Shift your attention to your lower legs. Feel the muscles in your shins and calves relaxing and getting so heavy it feels as though they're sinking into the mattress beneath them.

7. Slowly shift your attention up to each part of your body: your knees, thighs, buttocks, hips, stomach, lower back, upper back, shoulders, arms, hands, neck and head. Each time, imagine the muscles growing heavy and relaxed after a long day, and feel them fully supported by the mattress beneath your body.

8. Now that your body feels completely heavy and relaxed, return your attention to your breath. Don't attempt to change your breath at all; simply follow the pattern of your breath, gently focusing your attention on each inhale and exhale. If your attention slips, don't worry – simply shift your attention back to the breath.

9. Do this for as long as feels comfortable – perhaps until you drift off to sleep.

10. If you don't fall asleep following this meditation, don't worry – this is perfectly natural. Simply enjoy the sensation of feeling completely relaxed.

GETTING BACK TO SLEEP

Many people who suffer with sleep disruption can get to sleep easily enough – the problem is staying asleep. If you wake in the night, these anxiety first-aid tips might help you get back to sleep:

+ Avoid clock-watching: this can increase feelings of anxiety that you aren't asleep when you "should" be.

+ Avoid screens: blue light tricks your brain into thinking it's daytime.

+ Think about something dull: research conducted in 2018 found that when people focused on things they found boring, they felt sleepier.

+ Try a sleep meditation (page 70).

+ If something's on your mind, such as a task for the next day, jot it down on a piece of paper. This allows your mind to "forget" about it.

+ If you're still awake after 15 minutes, get out of bed and sit quietly for a few minutes. This can help you feel sleepier.

INHALE PEACE AND CALM, EXHALE STRESS AND ANXIETY

FEAR OF FAILURE, REJECTION AND CRITICISM

There's no easy way around it: failure, rejection and criticism suck. However, if you're so scared of failing – or being rejected or criticized – that you've stopped truly living, are no longer applying for dream jobs, entering competitions or trying anything new, then that's a problem.

Fear of failure is common and when it's chronic, it is known as – atychiphobia. With strong links to fears of criticism and rejection, it is also related to perfectionism – feeling like you shouldn't do anything unless it's absolutely perfect. And perfectionism is closely linked with – you guessed it – anxiety.

If fear of failure, rejection or criticism is holding you back, you might feel there's not much you can do about it. However, on pages 75, 78 and 79, we'll explore some powerful first-aid tips to help you understand where this fear comes from and how you can move beyond it.

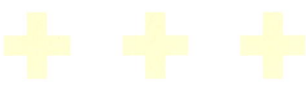

HOW TO GET GOOD AT FAILURE AND REJECTION

If you've avoided situations where you can fail or get rejected for a long time, the thought of it can be almost paralyzing. Engineering safe, low-stakes scenarios in which you can practise getting gentle knock-backs can be beneficial, to prove life goes on after failure and rejection – and you can even thrive afterward!

To get good at failure and rejection, you have to start trying new things and putting yourself out there. Remember, the whole point is failing at first – if you fail, that's great! A good place to start is to try learning a fun but challenging new skill or creative endeavour – think slacklining, juggling, hula-hooping, painting a landscape or writing a poem. Perhaps you could enter your painting or poem into a competition? You might not win, but who cares? You've been brave and that's what's important.

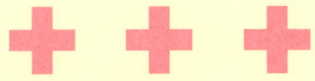

WHERE DO THESE FEARS STEM FROM?

Fears of failure, rejection and criticism can have many different causes. Some have deep roots, trailing back to past trauma. For example, if you were bullied as a child, any experience of criticism or rejection is likely to bring back these painful memories.

Fears of failure, criticism and rejection can often be linked to embarrassment, shame and feelings of not being good enough. These feelings are highly uncomfortable, so fear and anxiety kick in to try to protect us from ever having to experience them.

Then, there's the deep ancestral reason for these fears. In the past, if our early ancestors were rejected, criticized or failed at something, it might have led to them being ostracized, compromising their survival. Therefore, conforming and being seen to be doing well has become "safe".

The trouble is, feeling unable to express yourself, go for opportunities or live the way *you* want to means keeping yourself small, when really you are here to dream big, be yourself and thrive! Research shows that fear of failure can significantly hold you back, both professionally and personally. In fact, one study of 1,000 people, carried out by researchers from Nyenrode Business University and IE University, found that one in two people feel like they could perform better at work if they were not anxious about making mistakes. But if this sounds familiar, fear not! The following pages will provide some anxiety first aid designed to help you step out from under fear's shadow and live the way *you* want!

FIRST AID TO OVERCOME FEARS OF FAILURE AND REJECTION

If you struggle with this, the following first-aid strategies can help you begin to live a richer, fuller life:

+ Remember, everyone who's great at something has been rejected or failed – probably multiple times.

+ Reframe failure in your mind: failing is how you get good enough to finally succeed.

+ Allow yourself to be a beginner – no one is great at anything instantly. So adopt a beginner's mindset (having an open, curious outlook, as though you're approaching a task for the first time), put your perfectionism to one side and allow yourself to take small steps and make mistakes – it's how you'll grow.

+ Speak to people you view as "successful". Learning how many times they've failed, or been rejected or criticized, can help you view success as a learning curve, with multiple ups and downs along the way.

- Recognize the cost of not going for your dream. Consider the famous quote by Suzy Kassem: "Fear kills more dreams than failure ever will." In other words, by letting fear run the show, you'll end up never even trying. Sure, you'll never fail, be rejected or get criticized either... but at what cost? Isn't it time to step out of your comfort zone, try, fail, try again... and maybe start living your dream on the road to success?

- If anxiety is paralyzing you, try journalling as a way of unravelling your fears. What's really stopping you? Writing can help you discover those underlying thought patterns and anxieties, such as fear of embarrassment.

- Shift your mindset: if you're constantly worried about what others think, it's time to start forgetting about them and focusing on yourself instead. In other words, shifting from external to internal validation. Over the page, we'll take you through the steps to guide you.

HOW TO SHIFT FROM EXTERNAL TO INTERNAL VALIDATION

Feeling anxious about what people think of you, or waiting for the approval of others, can be frustrating, stressful and mentally draining. If this sounds familiar, it's likely you're relying heavily on external validation. This can happen when you regularly experience feelings of low self-worth, when you lack faith in your own ideas, opinions or choices, and when you are highly self-critical. All of this can result in high levels of anxiety, as you're constantly second-guessing what others want or what might make them happy, as opposed to focusing on what it is *you* want or what will make *you* happy. If you'd like to shift from external to internal validation (that is, honouring and appreciating your own values, qualities and opinions), here are some first-aid tips for you:

+ Practise mindfulness (see page 38). This can help shift your attention away from others, helping to still your mind and centre your focus on yourself in the moment.

- Harness the power of affirmations. Speaking kindly to yourself can do wonders for your self-esteem – you're literally "affirming" your own existence by repeating them. Phrases such as "I'm perfect exactly as I am" can really lift you up.

- Try journalling. Putting your thoughts and feelings down on paper can help you make sense of them and lead you to the answers you've been seeking, without the need to ask others for reassurance. Often, you intuitively know what's right for you.

- Get comfortable saying no to others (more on page 114). Often, if we fear rejection or criticism, we say yes to all requests, accommodating everyone else's happiness at the expense of our own. Putting yourself first sometimes by honouring your own needs is an important step to weaning yourself off external validation.

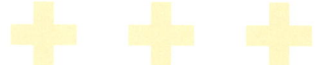

CHAPTER THREE:

SOCIAL SITUATIONS

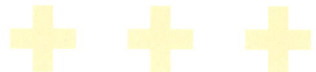

Many people without anxiety disorders still find certain social situations stressful. From giving a presentation to a room full of strangers or making small talk with your boss, to leaving a voicemail, going to the gym for the first time or heading on a date with someone you really like, there are loads of scenarios that can get our hearts racing and our mouths feeling dry. And if you suffer with social anxiety, these situations can feel excruciating. This chapter is packed with top tips and soothing advice to help you get through any number of anxiety-inducing social situations, leaving you feeling calmer, clearer-headed and more in control when you're out and about.

MEETING NEW PEOPLE

Whether it's at college, work or a party, meeting new people can be nerve-racking. For many, fears that we won't be liked or that people will find us boring swim round our brains. If you have social anxiety, meeting new people can be particularly fear-inducing, so much so that you might start avoiding new places and situations. If this sounds familiar, take a deep breath and read on – below are some anxiety first-aid tips to help take the fear out of meeting new people.

+ Plan ahead: have conversation starters planned. These could be about weekend plans or a movie you've seen recently.

+ Ask questions: asking others about themselves is a nice way to start a conversation and takes the focus away from you.

+ Identify triggers: what is it about meeting new people that you find hard? Is it starting a conversation, eating in front of others or using a public bathroom when others are around? It's easier to manage your anxiety when you understand your triggers.

- Remember, the focus isn't all on you, whatever your mind tells you! The reality is, everyone else is mostly just focused on themselves, too!

- Counteract negative thoughts such as "I'm so boring", "I'll embarrass myself" and "What if no one likes me?" Remind yourself these are just negative thoughts, then replace them with something more positive and realistic. For example: "I'm nervous, but I'm interesting and fun to be around."

- Introduce yourself to just a few people rather than telling yourself you have to mingle with everyone – this can take the pressure off.

- Tell yourself you'll stay for just half an hour. This can make the event seem more manageable and, if it starts going well, you can always stay longer!

MAKING NEW FRIENDS

Like meeting new people, making friends can be a daunting task. If you struggle because your anxiety plunges you into all sorts of negative thought spirals, here are some tips to help take the pressure off:

+ Remind yourself of your good qualities – maybe you're a great listener, find it easy to make people laugh or are empathetic. When you focus on all the things you like about yourself, these are more likely to come across to your potential new friend.

+ Ask questions: as with meeting new people in any situation, asking questions is a great icebreaker and takes the spotlight off you for a while. Remember to listen, rather than worrying about what you might say next!

+ If you're not sure where to meet like-minded people, think about what you love doing, then find a group or class to join. Doing an activity alongside others is a great way to take the pressure off, plus if they're at the class too, you know you already have a common interest!

- Take it slowly: remember, friendships take time. Meeting someone for coffee a few times won't instantly transform them into your BFF – and that's normal. Friendships are based on a whole host of factors, such as common interests, a shared sense of humour and trust, and these things can't be forced or developed overnight. Give it time!

- Take the pressure off: if a new friendship doesn't go anywhere, you haven't "failed". As with romantic relationships, not everyone is always compatible, so if a friendship fizzles out, commend yourself for having been brave enough to put yourself out there.

HOW TO START CONVERSATIONS

If all this talk of meeting new people and making friends has got you wondering "but *how* do I get started?", check out these icebreakers, perfect for a whole host of situations. These may come in handy where "small talk" is required – something many people feel anxious about, as it usually means conversing with people you may not know all that well. These conversation starters are almost guaranteed to get an interesting chat going… and they're certainly more thought-provoking than your average small talk about the weather!

"What's the most adventurous thing you've ever done?"

This is a great opener that will help you discover someone's values, likes and lust for life, and help you find out if you're compatible with them – if their answer is bungee jumping over a river in Australia and you're an adrenaline junkie, you're onto a winner!

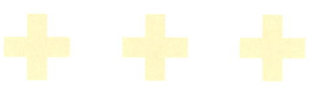

"What's something you used to do that you once thought was embarrassing but now think is cool?"

This one gives you an insight into a person's vulnerabilities in an offhand way – it might have you both opening up about the past or reminiscing about childhood fads or hairstyles!

"What's the last song you heard that made you get up and dance or sing out loud?"

This gives you an insight into whether the person is an introvert or extrovert and what music they listen to. Were they at a gig or having a solo kitchen disco? Alone or with friends? There's so much scope for a longer conversation with this one!

"If you could choose any superpower, what would it be?"

A silly question that can get you both thinking about your values or how you might want to change the world!

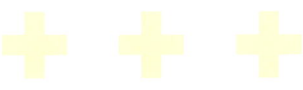

PUBLIC SPEAKING

Fear of speaking in public is a common source of anxiety, with symptoms ranging from mild nerves to outright panic. It will likely manifest as a racing pulse, dry mouth, trembling hands, shaky voice and brain fog – all things that are totally unhelpful for talking in front of a group of people! If this sounds familiar, these practical anxiety first-aid tips might help to calm your nerves:

+ Get organized: with public speaking, organization is key! If you can, visit the space you'll be speaking in and ask what tech or equipment will be available. If you struggle to memorize your presentation, make notes you can refer to.

+ Practise: then practise again… and again! Ask a friend or family member to be your audience and provide constructive feedback – or perhaps record yourself presenting so you can watch yourself back (this can also be anxiety-inducing, but check out our tips about overcoming camera shyness on page 54).

- Breathe deeply: a few mindful breaths can help to calm your nerves by regulating your sympathetic nervous system. Before you're introduced at your speaking engagement, pause and take a couple of deep breaths, inhaling fully through your nose until your belly expands, then exhaling deeply.

- Use visualization: before your presentation, visualize it going well. Picture how you'll feel, what you'll see and what you'll hear (applause from the audience at the end, perhaps). Doing a few mental rehearsals will help set you up for success.

- Focus on the content, not the audience: remember, your audience is listening because you have something interesting to share. So, focus your attention on what you're delivering, rather than worrying about how you're being perceived. Despite what you might think, the audience probably can't tell you're nervous and, even if they can, they'll be rooting for you.

SPEAKING ON THE PHONE

Many people get nervous about speaking on the phone (telephonophobia). Some dislike the sound of their own voice, while others struggle to pick up on verbal cues or feel uncomfortable making decisions in the moment. If you'd like some anxiety first aid to help you feel more confident on the phone, we have the tips for you!

+ Call a friend or loved one: to move beyond your fear, you have to get used to making phone calls! Start by calling someone you know for a quick chat.

+ Make notes: if you're worried you're going to forget to ask something important or run out of things to say, jot down a few notes you can refer to while speaking. Don't script the entire thing – this can make you sound too rehearsed and end up making you even more anxious – but a few bullet points can help you maintain your focus.

+ Smile! Even though the person on the end of the line can't see your facial expressions, smiling can lower your cortisol levels, helping you feel more relaxed.

How to leave a confident voicemail

For some, leaving a voicemail or voice note is even worse than chatting on the phone! Check out these tips to help keep your anxiety in check if you have to leave a message:

+ If a call goes to voicemail and you're caught off guard, it's fine to hang up, plan what you want to say clearly and concisely, and then call back when you're prepared.

+ Speak clearly and slowly.

+ Don't forget the essentials – your name, number and why you're calling.

+ As with making calls, start by leaving voicemails or voice notes for people you know well to help you get in the habit.

NAVIGATING SOCIAL MEDIA AND FOMO

Social media can be a fun, creative and inspiring platform for connecting with others and sharing opinions and ideas. However, it can also be highly addictive, due to the dopamine hit it provides, and it can also be bad for your mental health, fuelling anxiety, depression and self-doubt. If you frequently find yourself on social media worrying that others are having rewarding, fulfilling experiences while you're not, you may be suffering from "fear of missing out" (FOMO).

The anxiety caused by FOMO is very real and can lead to incessant scrolling through social media in search of more and more connections. It can have you interrupting one online chat to start another and checking your phone while in the company of friends, family or even while at work to make sure you don't "miss out". Of course, the reality is that FOMO and excessive social media use can result in pushing people close to you away as you favour multiple online chats or scrolling for meaningful one-to-one connection.

If social media and FOMO are damaging your mental health, try the following for some instant anxiety first-aid relief:

+ Talk to someone you trust about how social media is making you feel.

+ Schedule in some screen-free time each day – even just half an hour away from your phone can help.

+ Instead of scrolling, spend time doing things that make you feel happy, relaxed and content, such as going for a walk or meeting a friend for a coffee. In short, try swapping FOMO for JOMO (the "joy of missing out").

GOING SHOPPING

Whether it's a trip to the supermarket, shopping centre or high street, shopping can increase stress if you struggle with social anxiety. From the crowds of people, to the endless choice, to the sensory overload due to the bright lighting, noise and strong smells, even the thought of hitting the shops can be too much. Here are some first-aid tips to help you keep your cool when out and about:

+ Plan ahead: write a list of what you need to buy so you are not overwhelmed in the shop.

+ Go at an off-peak time: heading out when it's less busy might help you feel calmer.

+ Ask a friend to accompany you: going with a trusted companion can give you the moral support you need.

+ Try relaxation techniques: a breathing exercise (page 36) or the 3-3-3 technique (page 44) can help to keep you calm, present and focused.

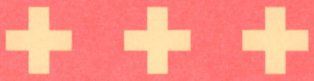

It's good to do uncomfortable things. It's weight training for life.

ANNE LAMOTT

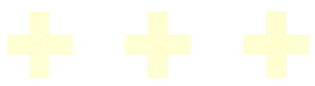

EATING IN PUBLIC

The fear of eating in front of others is known as deipnophobia. It can be a highly distressing form of social anxiety, and coping with it from day to day can be restrictive when it comes to socializing.

While anyone can experience deipnophobia, some people are at a higher risk of experiencing it. These higher-risk groups include:

+ People who currently have (or have previously had) an eating disorder.
+ People who are overweight (as they can feel judged by others).
+ People who have experienced abuse or coercive control (as eating can be seen as an intimate act, which can therefore be highly triggering for someone recovering from these experiences).

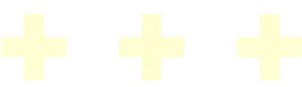

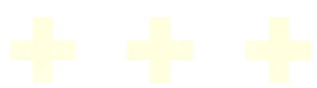

Because anxiety around food can have so many complex causes and triggers, treatment is not a simple one-size-fits-all solution. In fact, professional therapy is advised if this is something you struggle with. While feeling anxious about eating in front of others can be highly upsetting and you might feel you'll never move beyond it, cognitive behavioural therapy (CBT) and exposure therapy are often very effective. If you think you might benefit, it's important to contact your doctor.

For a spot of anxiety first aid in the moment, breathing exercises (page 36), the 3-3-3 technique (page 44), mindfulness (page 38) and meditation (page 40) can all be beneficial, but specialist support (as mentioned above) is important.

FEAR OF DRIVING

Feeling anxious about driving can be caused by a number of emotional and psychological factors. These can include:

+ Past trauma, such as an accident, incident or altercation.

+ Fear of having an accident, losing control or making a mistake.

+ Aversion to driving anywhere new or unfamiliar.

+ Not knowing where to park upon arrival.

Overcoming driving anxiety can seem daunting, and professional support in the form of CBT or exposure therapy can be beneficial. However, there are some first-aid measures you can take to help ease your fears:

+ Identify your specific triggers: is it driving in heavy traffic or on motorways, navigating city centres, concerns about parking or getting lost, or something else? Pinpointing your exact worries can make driving seem less overwhelming.

+ Bring a companion: having a friend or family member in the passenger seat can give you extra support and confidence, plus they can help you out with navigation if you get stuck.

+ Use relaxation techniques: a breathing exercise or short meditation before you head off can work wonders to help keep your nerves under control.

+ Try visualization: visualizing your journey beforehand can help you prepare mentally and emotionally. As you go through your visualization, imagine yourself feeling calm, happy and confident as you're driving.

+ Repeat affirmations: if you feel your anxiety starting to rise, trying repeating a short, empowering mantra: "I am in control", "I am safe" or "I am competent" can serve as helpful reminders.

+ Start small: be patient with yourself as you build your confidence and start with short local journeys.

GOING TO THE GYM

Heading for a gym session can present all manner of opportunities for anxiety, from worrying you don't know how to use the equipment correctly to "imposter syndrome" (thinking you don't fit in there). If you struggle with going to the gym, try these anxiety first-aid tips:

+ Remember, you have just as much right to be in the gym as everyone else. Everyone was a beginner once!

+ Consider a personal trainer session: if you don't know your way around the equipment, a session with an expert can develop your knowledge and boost your confidence.

+ Focus on your own goals, rather than what others are doing. Comparing yourself with someone else is counterproductive – you don't know what their goals are or how long they've been training for.

+ Remember, no one is looking at you as much as you think they are!

ONLINE DATING AND FIRST-DATE ANXIETY

Setting up an online dating profile or joining a dating app is nerve-racking for everyone. It's the same when going on a date: even the most confident of people feel anxious because putting yourself out there makes you feel vulnerable. Dating involves exposing yourself to potential rejection and (gulp) shame. BUT... just because it's scary doesn't mean it's something you should shy away from! While it's nerve-racking, having the courage to be honest, open and vulnerable with someone new is the way to start forming a genuine connection. Over the following pages, you'll find anxiety first-aid tips to help you navigate both the online dating world and in-person first dates with a little more confidence.

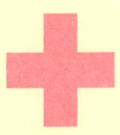

ANXIETY FIRST AID FOR DATING

Joining a dating app

+ Your profile doesn't need to be perfect: remember, the profile isn't the end result – it's merely the icebreaker. You don't need to prove that you're the cleverest, wittiest person out there; it just needs to give an accurate picture of you – including any unique quirks – to help you on your way to genuine connection.

+ Be honest: there's no point trying to play it cool by listing hobbies and interests you think make you sound great but that you have no real interest in. Remember, the whole point is to find someone you gel with, so if you have an unusual interest or pastime, mention it!

+ Share what you're looking for: if you're looking for a meaningful, long-lasting relationship, say so! This will stop you having to feel anxious about fielding those who are after something more casual. It's the same the other way round: there's no shame in not wanting a serious relationship, but be honest about this so that you meet like-minded people.

Going on a first date

+ Reframe the first date in your mind: it's not an interview, it's an adventure!

+ Remember, your date is nervous too: knowing you're both in the same boat can help ease your anxiety.

+ Be honest: if you're feeling shy or extremely nervous, let them know! Being open can help break the ice and get you laughing together.

+ Ask questions: remember, as with meeting new people and making friends (page 86), if you hate being in the spotlight, ask questions. This will shift the focus off you for a while, giving you space to relax.

COPING WITH INTIMACY OR SEXUAL ANXIETY

If you experience anxiety when it comes to getting intimate with someone else, be it a new or long-term partner, you're not alone. In fact, according to a 2020 study published in *Sexual Medicine Reviews*, sexual performance anxiety is one of the most prevalent sexual complaints, affecting up to 25 per cent of men and 16 per cent of women.

Anxiety relating to sex and intimacy can stem from many causes, including past sexual abuse, body image issues, relationship issues, overthinking during sex and incompatibility with your partner. If sexual anxiety is something you struggle with, there's nothing to be ashamed of, and if it has its roots in trauma, it's important to seek professional support from a qualified therapist who can help you work through trust and intimacy issues in a safe environment. There are, however, some anxiety first-aid tips that can help, too. You could try the following:

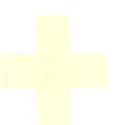

- Talk to your partner. This might seem obvious, but it can be a difficult yet vital first step. Speaking openly and honestly can make the subject feel less pressured.
- Remember, intimacy isn't just about sex. Try initiating non-sexual touch with your partner, such as a massage, cuddling or hand-holding, to increase feelings of intimacy without any pressure.
- Get to know your own body, as well as your own likes and dislikes, through masturbation.
- When getting intimate, take the pressure off by agreeing things don't have to lead to sex. Simply spend time having fun together!

DEALING WITH CONFLICT

In an ideal world, we'd never have to deal with conflict. Sadly, though, conflict is part of life because everyone is different, with their own (sometimes conflicting) ideas and opinions. From online altercations and people ignoring your boundaries (more on page 110), to work conflicts, relationship disagreements and even misunderstandings with strangers in the supermarket queue, most of us will encounter conflict from time to time.

If the thought of getting into a conflict brings you out in a cold sweat, remember, it doesn't have to involve harsh words. Staying calm can work wonders.

Let's take an example of someone who constantly disregards your opinion at work. If the thought of confronting them makes your anxiety spiral to the point where you avoid the issue, they will likely just keep at it – which will damage your self-confidence and make you feel worse in the long run. So, it's time to be brave, let them know and set a boundary regarding their behaviour. You could take them to one side and explain your grievance in a clear, calm way. You could also offer a consequence if they continue the behaviour after you've spoken about it. Your chat could go something like this: "We spoke about the fact I don't feel you listen to me or take my suggestions on board. But you still talk over me. If you continue to do so in future, I'm going to end the meeting."

Your scenario might look different to this, but good rules of thumb for handling conflict include:

1. Stay calm and speak clearly, without raising your voice.
2. Be clear in your intentions.
3. Set a boundary if necessary.
4. State the consequence if your boundary continues to be ignored.

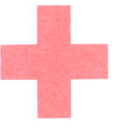

WHY BOUNDARIES ARE IMPORTANT

If you struggle with anxiety, boundaries protect your time and energy, giving you the space you need to rest and relax – and this is vital when it comes to managing stress. Setting clear and effective boundaries could (and should!) form a key part of your anxiety first-aid kit. Boundaries in social settings could look like:

+ Turning down a request to take on a project at work.
+ Declining a social invitation that you genuinely don't want to attend.
+ Explaining to others that you won't be drinking alcohol at a work or social event.

As you can see, setting boundaries often involves letting others down for the sake of your own mental health. This is hard, but necessary… and we'll explore how to get comfortable with it over the following pages.

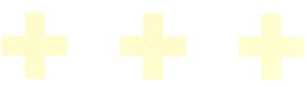

PAUSE, BREATHE AND BELIEVE IN YOURSELF

HOW TO SET EFFECTIVE BOUNDARIES

Boundaries are vital in all areas of life, from the workplace to social settings and relationships. Setting boundaries can seem difficult at first, especially if you usually make yourself readily available to everyone to the detriment of your own health, happiness and anxiety levels. But drawing a line to determine what is and isn't acceptable to you can reduce feelings of anxiety, as well as boost your self-esteem and well-being.

Identifying missing boundaries

Think about your relationships for a moment. Do any of them bring up feelings of anxiety, resentment, unease or anger? If so, it's possible the boundaries of your relationship with that person are unclear. Consider what might be causing an issue. For example, does the person in question disregard your personal space? Do they use you as an emotional sounding board without ever asking what's going on in your life? Do they expect favour after favour, without offering anything in return?

Identifying the boundary required is an important first step toward applying some anxiety first aid.

Putting a boundary in place

Once you've identified the problem, it's time to set the boundary. Think about a good time to establish it. During an argument isn't ideal; wait until you're both calm and have time to talk. Use "I" rather than "you" statements to prevent it from feeling accusatory, and be clear and specific. For example, instead of saying something vague like: "I need more time alone to relax and de-stress," you could try: "I love our time together, but I also need time for my own hobbies to help me unwind, and I know these don't interest you. I'm going to start dedicating Tuesday and Thursday evenings to these." A calm tone shows you're serious, while maintaining respect.

LEARNING THE ART OF SAYING NO

If you automatically say *yes* to requests without considering your own commitments, workload or mental well-being, you'll be on a fast track to heightened anxiety. This is why getting comfortable with *no* is such an important element of your anxiety first-aid kit. We often feel guilty for saying *no* because it can feel like a rejection of the other person. However, saying *yes* when you don't want to can lead to resentment, which is why saying *no* really can be the right thing to do.

Saying *no* doesn't have to be rude. A simple "thanks for asking, but I'm afraid I don't have space for that right now" or "I'd love to help, but unfortunately I'm already juggling multiple projects" are two firm but polite responses that will leave you feeling empowered, less overwhelmed and less anxious. Try not to fall into the trap of over-explaining yourself or apologizing profusely. After all, in saying *no*, you're doing nothing wrong.

Speaking up for yourself can be nerve-racking, so it's helpful to practise what you need to say first, before you do it for real. Here are some tips:

+ Write down key points to help you formulate your thoughts.

+ Use these notes to guide you as you speak the words out loud, either on your own or to a trusted friend.

+ Try out your new-found "speaking up for yourself" voice in a low-stakes situation first. For example, if you need to say *no* to a work request, practise saying *no* to something easier first, such as a social invite you want to turn down.

+ Remember, practice makes perfect – and it will show you nothing bad comes from putting your own needs first sometimes.

HOW TO OVERCOME LEADERSHIP ANXIETY

Not every leader operates with self-assuredness and confidence. Having to manage others can often cause anxiety, especially if you're new to a leadership position.

Leadership anxiety can be caused by a number of factors, including nerves about telling others what to do, worries about letting people down and fears you're not qualified enough for the role ("imposter syndrome"). Below, you'll find some key leadership anxiety first aid to help you out when you're in the spotlight and the pressure's on at work.

+ Communicate clearly: if you're nervous in your leadership role, be honest about this! Letting your team know that you're new and that you're finding your feet can sometimes be a great icebreaker. If this level of vulnerability doesn't feel appropriate, it's still important to be honest with your team. If they ask for guidance and you're unsure of the way forward, never lie by making something up: simply tell them you'll get back to them to give yourself a little research time.

- Seek out a mentor: seeking guidance from someone else in a senior position can be a great way to learn the ropes and gain confidence if you're anxious. Is there someone you admire who you can invite for coffee so you can chat about leadership tips and management style?

- Believe in yourself: imposter syndrome (the belief that you aren't good enough and have been given a role by mistake, which might lead to being "found out") can feel very real. If this is something you struggle with, remember you have been given this role for a reason. Others believe in you – now it's time for you to start believing in yourself. If you're finding the transition to leadership tough, you could request specific leadership training to help ease your anxieties.

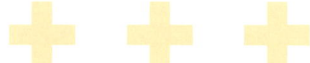

CHAPTER FOUR:

THE WIDER WORLD

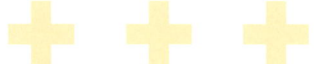

Over the previous chapters, we've taken an in-depth look at some of the reasons why you might feel anxious in relation to personal and social issues. But of course, external factors can also heavily influence our anxiety levels and emotional state. These can range from specific situations and stressors, such as work pressure, deadlines, exams and financial worries, to wider global issues, such as eco-anxiety, political anxiety and other distressing events we witness in the news each day. In this chapter, we'll look at various ways in which the wider world can impact our anxiety and the measures we can take to protect our mental and emotional health.

COPING WITH CHANGE

Big life changes bring with them feelings of uncertainty and anxiety. This is because anxiety often stems from fear of the unknown, including worries about future events over which we have no control. We also have no way of knowing whether a life change will be a success, so our brains naturally tend to go into overdrive, cycling through every possible outcome and usually hyper-fixating on the negatives.

Your big life change might be something you've instigated yourself and are excited about. But even so, anxiety and fear will both still find ways of creeping in and spoiling the party. Examples of positive life changes that can cause anxiety include:

+ Heading to college or university.
+ Moving house, especially if it's to a new area.
+ Going travelling.
+ Starting a new job.
+ Having children.

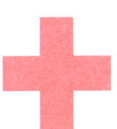

Sometimes we'll go through a big life change that we never wanted to happen. Examples of these include:

+ Being made redundant.
+ Separation or divorce.
+ The death of a loved one.

Over the next few pages, we'll take a closer look at some of these changes, examining the specific triggers involved and identifying ways to help you cope, which you can add to your anxiety first-aid kit.

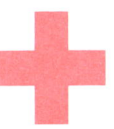

HEADING TO COLLEGE OR UNIVERSITY

Moving away from home to attend college or university can be daunting. On the one hand, you're entering an exciting new period of your life, filled with opportunities to meet lots of new people and have new experiences, and yet, on the other, you may be leaving behind all that is safe and familiar. The pressure to make new friends and have fun can bring with it anxiety, while worries about not "fitting in" have the potential to increase feelings of insecurity. While this time of your life is billed as an exciting chance to experience independence, it's perfectly normal to feel anxious about it. Leaving family, close friends and home comforts behind can be hard, and the shock to your system can make you want to hide away in your room outside of lectures and seminars. Here are a few coping mechanisms that might help you manage the transition:

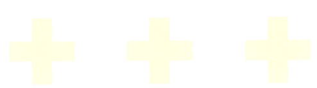

- If you're struggling to adapt, remind yourself you're not the only one! Simply knowing that others are sharing your feelings can make you feel less anxious and alone.

- If you're struggling to meet new people, try joining a club, group or society that interests you. This way, you know the other people there will have similar interests to you.

- If social anxiety is overwhelming you, break it down into a more manageable task: telling yourself you'll just try and speak to one new person in the common room, kitchen or after a lecture can boost your confidence.

- If your anxiety is stopping you have the experience you'd like, seek support from student counselling services.

MOVING HOME

Moving back home can cause as much stress and anxiety as moving away. After all, it's a big commitment and huge change that can bring uncertainty, which anxiety thrives on. Remember, it's natural to feel anxious at times like this, but this simple technique can help you feel less overwhelmed:

"Close the loop"

You have so much to think about when moving home, including calling solicitors, transferring money, booking removal vans and packing, so whenever you remember something, add it to a to-do list. This technique is called "closing the loop": even though you haven't done the task yet, writing it down tells your brain you can forget about it for now, so it stops swirling round your head in an endless loop. You can attend to it when it's time to perform the task. This works for other situations, too, when you have lots to remember.

BEING MADE REDUNDANT

Being out of work – whether expected or unexpected – is a big change, which can bring with it feelings of anxiety. If you've spent much of your adult life performing a particular role in society, suddenly being unable to do that can create a sense of loss. If you find yourself out of work, regularly engaging with the practices explored in Chapter One can help, including mindfulness (page 38), meditation (page 40) and breathwork (page 36). You might also find the tips on dealing with financial anxiety (page 138) helpful. While you're out of work, you could seek out voluntary or charitable opportunities – after all, helping others is one of the best antidotes to anxiety, as you shift your focus off yourself and onto others (more on page 150). Volunteering can also give you sense of purpose and connection, and might even lead to future employment.

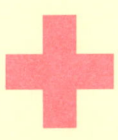

BEREAVEMENT, GRIEF AND ANXIETY

The death of a loved one is most often associated with feelings of grief and sadness, but it can also come with other emotions. Anxiety is an often-overlooked reaction to grief, but it's a perfectly normal response.

Being confronted with death can prompt us to consider our own mortality, which can be highly uncomfortable, and the death of someone close to us can put us under significant stress, especially if we're responsible for making funeral arrangements or sorting through the person's belongings – both of which can make us feel emotionally vulnerable. If the person's death was expected, for example if they were suffering from a terminal illness, you will likely have experienced considerable anxiety in the run-up to their passing, especially if you had to take on caring duties.

If you're experiencing anxiety as part of grieving, be gentle with yourself. These ideas might provide some relief while you mourn:

- Try journalling: writing down your thoughts and feelings can help you untangle and make sense of them.
- Try the 3-3-3 technique on page 44: this can help to ground you in the present in moments when your anxiety and grief begin to spiral.
- Take a moment for a short meditation or breathing exercise: these can help to calm you.
- Talk to someone: sharing your feelings with a friend, family member, someone who has been through a bereavement or a trained grief counsellor is important if you're struggling.

WORK-RELATED ANXIETY

Workplace stress and anxiety have become so commonplace that many people believe they are normal. But it doesn't have to be this way and, if you're struggling, there are steps you can take to help you feel calmer.

What causes workplace anxiety?

Anxiety in the workplace can have numerous causes. If you've started a new job, it's normal to feel nervous about meeting a new team of people and settling into a new workplace and routine. However, if the anxiety persists for more than a few weeks, there might be something more going on. Perhaps a form of social anxiety makes you anxious about giving a presentation, speaking up in a meeting, dealing with clients or customers, or working directly with senior leaders. Maybe you're struggling with deadlines or managing your work–life balance, or perhaps there's a particular colleague who triggers your anxiety.

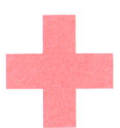

Symptoms of workplace anxiety

The symptoms of workplace anxiety are similar to those of other forms of anxiety, including a racing pulse, feelings of nausea and excessive sweating. However, workplace anxiety can also have some unique symptoms. These include:

+ Feeling like you need to be perfect.
+ Losing interest in your work.
+ Needing days off due to poor mental health and anxiety.
+ Making mistakes and struggling to fulfil your duties.

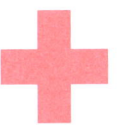

COPING WITH ANXIETY AT WORK

If you're struggling with workplace anxiety, there are strategies that can help you. As well as the usual mindfulness techniques, breathwork and adopting healthy habits, such as getting enough sleep and eating well (which are beneficial for all forms of anxiety), there are a few additional techniques you can add to your anxiety first-aid kit, which can be applied in a workplace setting:

+ Set clear boundaries: for example, make sure you take your full lunch break to de-stress daily and don't take work home with you.

+ Avoid toxic colleagues: are you triggered by office gossip or negativity? Then steer clear.

+ Seek support: many workplaces now have designated mental health first-aiders, who you can chat to confidentially.

+ Communicate with managers: it's important to tell senior leaders if you're struggling. They might not realize the pressure you've been under.

If you don't like something, change it. If you can't change it, change your attitude.

MAYA ANGELOU

STUDY-RELATED ANXIETY

Studying at school, college or university can be stressful. Keeping up with assignments, managing deadlines, revising for exams and maintaining a social life is a lot to juggle. Here are some first-aid tips to help you keep your cool. You'll also find specific information about managing deadlines and handling exam pressure over the following pages:

+ Make sure you're looking after all aspects of your health, including eating healthily, getting enough sleep and not drinking too much alcohol. A balanced lifestyle can help with your mental health.

+ Try relaxation techniques, such as mindfulness and breathing exercises.

+ Talk to a friend or tutor about how you're feeling.

+ Calmly plan ahead where possible – for example, create a revision timetable so you have plenty of time to prepare without feeling rushed.

+ Try to stay organized – keeping an assignment diary can be helpful, so you know you won't miss any important deadlines.

HOW TO HANDLE DEADLINES

Deadlines can loom large in both your student life and at work. Some people thrive under the pressure of a deadline, while others struggle to stay focused, instead procrastinating or prioritizing the wrong things and ending up feeling stressed and anxious. If this sounds familiar, don't worry – try these three tips designed to help you handle deadlines with ease:

+ Create a checklist: set out everything you need to have completed by the deadline, then prioritize the toughest tasks first.

+ Set yourself "fake" deadlines: telling yourself you must have everything completed a few days early might sound like putting even more pressure on yourself, but it can actually take the pressure off in the long run.

+ Take regular short breaks: no one can work at full throttle all day, every day. Factor in short relaxation breaks.

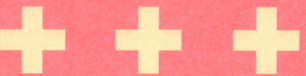

TAKING EXAMS

Exam anxiety is a very specific type of stress. When studying for (and taking) exams, it's important to remember that a certain amount of stress is a good thing. This is known as "eustress" and it helps to focus your mind on the task at hand, keeping you fired up and energized for revision. However, if your anxiety levels get too high, they can have an adverse effect, leading to panic, the inability to concentrate, headaches and stomach cramps. If you struggle with exam anxiety, here are a few practical anxiety first-aid tips that can help you keep your cool under pressure:

+ Revise in a way that suits you: that could be at home or in a library, alone or in a group, making notes or reciting lines as you go for a walk.

+ Make a timetable: planning what you have to do and when can take the pressure off.

+ Take regular breaks: planning in adequate downtime will help you maintain focus in the long run. After all, no one concentrates well when they're burned out.

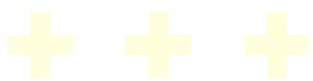

- Reframe your exam: it isn't there to catch you out, but instead is an opportunity to show off your knowledge.
- Get organized the night before your exam: make sure you have everything you'll need – and maybe bring a small "lucky" item with you, such as a special pen, badge or toy, for encouragement.
- Plan a rewarding activity for when your exams are over to give you something fun to look forward to.
- Remember, it's not the end of the world if things don't go to plan: everything will still be okay. You're still a wonderful, talented, unique individual, even if you fail an exam or two, so take the pressure off yourself and believe that everything will work out in the end.

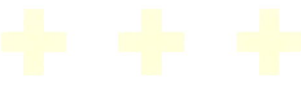

FINANCIAL ANXIETY

Money problems are a common source of anxiety, so if you're struggling with financial worries, know that you're not the only one. However insurmountable your situation may seem, there will be things you can do to help take the pressure off and ease your anxiety, so don't feel that it's hopeless – or that you have to go through it alone.

Causes of financial anxiety

While everyone's situation will be different, there are a few common factors that can contribute to financial anxiety. These include:

+ Debt, including loans, being in your overdraft or having maxed-out credit cards.

+ Feeling overwhelmed by bills or the monthly mortgage/rent.

+ Lack of savings or a "safety net", should unexpected expenses occur.

+ Periods of unemployment.

+ Having to manage an irregular income.

MONEY AND MENTAL HEALTH

Money worries and poor mental health are often intrinsically entwined, with one affecting the other and vice versa. For example, if you struggle with your mental health, this might lead to ignoring bills, putting off seeking financial advice, overspending as a way of trying to lift your mood, or struggling to hold down a job and therefore having to deal with employment uncertainty.

Conversely, financial worries can affect your mental health by causing anxiety or depression, feelings of guilt or shame, isolation and loneliness through having less money for socializing, and sleep problems.

As you can see, this pattern can become a vicious cycle, leading to a decline in mental health *and* financial security… which is why it's vital to apply some anxiety first aid to break the cycle!

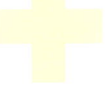

TIPS FOR TACKLING FINANCIAL ANXIETY

Take comfort from the fact that thousands of people have overcome money problems – and you can, too. Here's a step-by-step guide to tackling financial anxiety… and the great news? You can start right now:

1. First, stop ignoring any financial issues and hoping they will go away on their own. They won't. It's time to face them head on.

2. Talk to someone you trust. There can be a lot of shame attached to money problems, but there shouldn't be. Everyone struggles with money sometimes. Don't let stigma stop you getting support.

3. Call someone who can help. A financial support charity can help you start tackling your financial struggles. Similarly, make that call to the bank, mortgage lender, credit card company or utility provider. Letting them know you're struggling is important. They may be able to help, for example, by putting you on

a payment plan rather than expecting you to pay a bill in one lump sum.

4. Start paying off just one debt, even if it's only a small but regular amount. Getting started can ease your anxiety, helping you feel more in control.

5. Draw up a weekly budget – and stick to it. This will help you see where you can cut back and start saving.

6. If possible, aim to always have a buffer of three months' salary in your current account, in case of financial emergency.

7. Finally, anxiety around money is stressful, so do something nice for yourself each week that doesn't cost any money. Go for a walk in the fresh air, borrow a book from the library, invite a friend over for a chat or try some of the calming self-care ideas outlined in Chapter One, such as a meditation (page 40) or the 3-3-3 technique (page 44).

GLOBAL ANXIETY TRIGGERS

From climate change and political uncertainty, to news of wars, famines and terrorist activity, global issues and mass events can take their toll, heightening our anxiety and damaging our mental well-being. News of a crisis unfolding can be highly distressing. It can make us feel helpless in the face of a disaster happening elsewhere in the world, or can lead us to worry about a similar thing happening to those we love. A global disaster, such as the consequences of war for innocent civilians, can also trigger feelings of guilt – it can make us feel bad for being safe, secure and having nice things when others are suffering. Over the following pages, we'll look at ways in which you can protect your mental health in times of global uncertainty and upheaval, as well as ways you can empower yourself and turn your anxiety into positive action.

POLITICAL ANXIETY

Politics can be stressful. During periods of change and unrest, uncertainty can induce high levels of anxiety, and many people worry about the fate of themselves, their loved ones and specific communities in the event of a certain political outcome. Election campaigns can also cause divisive rifts through communities, social circles and even families, as people who we once felt aligned with socially take a different side or have different opinions to us. This can lead us to question our sense of belonging, which can be highly triggering and heighten our stress and anxiety.

Even if you take little interest in politics, this form of anxiety can reach you through community and social spaces. Over the page, we'll take a look at some ideas you can add to your anxiety first-aid kit to help manage this very specific type of anxiety.

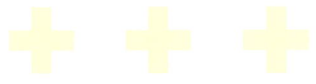

HOW TO HANDLE POLITICAL ANXIETY

Political anxiety can induce feelings of acute stress, especially around election times or when a candidate or political leader visits your region. To help you cope, there are steps you can take to help:

+ Limit your news consumption: with 24-hour coverage, we can feel a need to see every update as it breaks. But this isn't good for you, so switch off regularly.

+ Take a social media break: around election times, social media can get heated, vicious and toxic. Consider muting your accounts for a while.

+ Live your values: focus on what you can do by positively contributing to your community – for example, by helping a friend in need.

+ Take positive action: suggestions on pages 148–151 can help you channel your anxiety into a proactive response. Often, voting in elections also instils a sense of public spirit that helps to relieve anxiety.

YOU ARE STRONGER THAN YOU THINK

ANXIETY AND GLOBAL DISASTERS

From conflict, war and terrorist attacks to epidemics and natural disasters, adverse world events can be highly triggering, upsetting and anxiety-inducing. The anxiety that arises in the face of global disaster can feel all-consuming, but there are measures you can add to your anxiety first-aid kit to help you cope.

+ Sign up to a positive-only news outlet: of course it's important to stay up to date with events via traditional news reports, but accessing positive news stories as well can help you cultivate a more balanced world view. Remember, adding to your anxieties won't help you function well, and balancing your news consumption can help you to stay strong.

+ Curate your social media feed: now's not the time to engage with toxic, triggering posts. Instead, consider curating your feed to channel the power of people doing positive things. In a crisis, it's a good idea to focus on the helpers – the people, charities and organizations making a positive impact, so follow a few of these.

- Practise self-care: eat well, drink plenty of water, get out in the fresh air, exercise and aim for a good sleep every night. All these things can help you stay refreshed and feel more mentally resilient.

- Use relaxation techniques: practising relaxation, with meditation and breathwork, can help you stay calm amid global events.

- Ask for support: if you're struggling mentally, it's a good idea to ask for support – speak to friends, family or colleagues. Global disasters tend to have a widespread impact, and knowing you're not the only one struggling mentally can build a sense of community. If you're really struggling, you could contact a trained therapist.

ECO-ANXIETY AND PROACTIVE STEPS TO MANAGE IT

Eco-anxiety springs from feelings of uncertainty, helplessness and frustration in response to climate change. Many scientists and psychologists believe it's actually a healthy response to this threat – after all, climate change is something that affects us all. To manage eco-anxiety and ensure it doesn't harm your mental well-being, it's important to acknowledge its validity before finding ways to channel your worry, stress and anxiety through positive action. Taking practical steps can alleviate a sense of helplessness and you can bolster your anxiety first-aid kit by:

Making changes to your personal behaviour

Committing to live in a more environmentally friendly way is a great way to help combat eco-anxiety. There are so many small changes you can make to your lifestyle to ensure you're having as little negative impact on the planet as possible.

These include avoiding single-use plastic, eating less meat, using public transport instead of driving, buying second-hand clothes instead of new ones, reducing your food waste, buying locally grown produce, growing your own food, and recycling and reusing instead of throwing items away.

Joining an activist group or climate support network

Often, by joining other like-minded people, you can make a greater impact. Activist groups and networks organize rallies and protests, start petitions and draw attention to companies that pose the biggest climate threats in order to achieve change.

The idea is to reduce your anxiety by using it to fuel proactive, positive change. But of course, if you're really struggling, seeking professional anxiety treatments, such as CBT, can be an important step for your health and well-being.

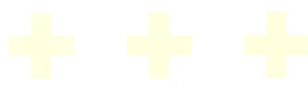

ACTIONS FOR COPING WITH GLOBAL ANXIETY TRIGGERS

With all global triggers, from political uncertainty and war to climate change and cultural shifts, harnessing your anxiety to fuel a positive, proactive response can be one of the best tools in your anxiety first-aid kit. Here are a few ideas to get you started:

Sign a petition

Sometimes, positive action can take as little as a minute – the time it takes to write your name on an online petition and click "add". If you're feeling anxious because of a particular issue, adding your name to (or even starting) a petition is a peaceful and powerful way to bring it to the attention of those in charge. Often, one voice won't make a difference, but the collective power of names on a petition can instigate positive change.

Write a letter

Writing a letter is another peaceful step you can take to help instigate change. If there's a local, political or climate-related issue that's making you anxious, writing to your local politician or representative is a way of bringing it to their attention and getting your voice heard.

Join (or organize!) a protest

Joining (or organizing) a peaceful protest is a powerful way to call for positive change and boost your mental health if you're struggling with global, political or environmental issues. Taking part in a march, sit-in or other demonstration alongside like-minded people can foster a sense of solidarity and community, which in itself can make the world feel a bit brighter. Peaceful protest is a human right, so if you feel the need to join the collective, don't be afraid to get out there!

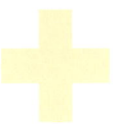

CHANNEL YOUR ENERGY INTO HELPING OTHERS

One of the best ways to relieve anxiety (whatever its cause) is to start putting your energy into something positive by helping others. Anxiety can leave us stuck inside the prison of our own minds, repeating worst-case scenarios over and over or only seeing the negatives in life. The solution, therefore, can be to start looking for the good – good things, people and causes that you can get involved with!

Research shows that those who spend time volunteering often report a strong sense of purpose (which can help alleviate anxiety), as well as increased happiness and confidence. So, is there a project, cause or campaign you care about that you could spare some time for? There are so many possibilities out there – you could help out at a food bank or soup kitchen, become a dementia befriender, support children's reading at a local school, volunteer at a wildlife sanctuary, help out with environmental clean-up in your area, volunteer at a museum or heritage site, or get stuck into a community gardening project. The options are almost endless! Check out community noticeboards or online groups to see where you can lend a hand. Even if you can only spare an hour a week, it will be time well spent, and knowing you're helping to make the world a little better can be the best way to counteract stress, sadness and anxiety.

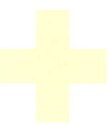

CONCLUSION

If you suffer with anxiety, you'll know the symptoms can be distressing and uncomfortable. But hopefully, by engaging with this book, you now feel less alone in your struggle and also know that, whatever the cause of your anxiety, there are steps you can take to help manage your symptoms and get your mental health back on track.

The purpose of this book is to provide some essential anxiety first aid for a range of scenarios and situations that might trigger feelings of anxiety and stress. So, whenever things get tough, why not flick back through these pages to find the relevant tips and techniques for whatever you're going through? There's a handy index on page 156, so you can quickly find the specific advice that will help you.

Of course, it's important to remember that this book is designed as first aid and contains strategies and advice to help when your anxiety is acute or when a certain event happens that you find challenging or triggering. If your anxiety is ongoing, or if the tips and techniques covered in this book don't seem to be having a significant impact for you, it's always important to seek the advice and support of a qualified therapist or practitioner. There are also some useful resources over the page to help when you're struggling. Hopefully, though, these words have had a positive impact on your mindset, and you can step into the next phase of your life feeling confident and anxiety-free.

RESOURCES

Books

Barnes, Anna *The Anxiety Fix* (2024, Vie): practical tips and simple strategies for managing anxiety.

Given, Florence *Women Living Deliciously* (2024, Brazen): move beyond your anxiety and internal barriers to live the life you deserve.

Haig, Matt *The Comfort Book* (2021, Canongate): a collection of suggestions to make bad days better.

O'Kane, Owen *Addicted to Anxiety* (2025, Michael Joseph): how to take back control from anxiety.

Websites and charities

988 Suicide & Crisis Lifeline: 24/7 free, confidential support for those in distress, as well as crisis resources for loved ones. www.988lifeline.org; 988 (USA)

Anxiety & Depression Association of America: education, training and research for anxiety, depression and related disorders. www.adaa.org (USA)

Anxiety UK: information, support and understanding for those living with anxiety disorders. www.anxietyuk.org.uk (UK)

Beat: support for those with eating disorders, as well as their loved ones. www.beateatingdisorders.org.uk (UK)

CALM: Campaign Against Living Miserably (CALM) is leading a movement against male suicide. www.thecalmzone.net (UK)

Freedom From Fear: a national non-profit mental health advocacy organization, helping to positively impact the lives of all those affected by anxiety, depression and related disorders. www.freedomfromfear.org (USA)

Mental Health America: promoting the overall mental health of all Americans. www.mhanational.org (USA)

Mental Health Foundation: a non-profit charitable organization specializing in mental health awareness, education, suicide prevention and addiction. www.mentalhealthfoundation.org (USA)

Mind: support and advice to help empower anyone experiencing a mental health problem. www.mind.org.uk (UK)

Samaritans: a 24-hour, free, confidential helpline to support you whatever you're going through. www.samaritans.org; 116 123; jo@samaritans.org (UK) / jo@samaritans.ie (Republic of Ireland)

Podcasts

Happy Place hosted by Fearne Cotton: conversations with inspirational people about life, loss and everything in-between.

Open with Emma Campbell: open-hearted conversations about life's challenges, including both the messy and magical bits.

Owning It: The Anxiety Podcast hosted by Caroline Foran: a practical and relaxed series exploring all aspects of anxiety.

10% Happier hosted by Dan Harris: learn how to make your life better, through mindfulness and meditation techniques.

We Can Do Hard Things hosted by Glennon Doyle, Abby Wambach and Amanda Doyle: getting through the hard things together, through open, enlightening conversations.

INDEX

A

Ageing 56–57
Alcohol/drug use 58–62
Anxiety, disorders 19
Anxiety, reframing 34–35
Anxiety, symptoms 13
Anxiety, triggers 16–17
Anxiety, what is it? 12

B

Bedtime routine 68–69
Bereavement 126–127
Breathing 36
Body dysmorphic disorder 50
Body image 48–49, 52–53
Boundaries 110–113

C

Comparison syndrome 27
Conflict 108–109
Coping strategies, an introduction 32
Coping with change 120–121
Criticism 74–79

D

Deadlines 133
Disordered eating 51

Driving, fear of 100–101

E

Eating disorders 51
Eating in public 98–99
Eco-anxiety 146–147

F

Fear of failure 74–79
Fight, flight or freeze response 15
Financial anxiety 136–139
First-date anxiety 103–105
FOMO 94–95

G

Generalized anxiety disorder 20
Getting back to sleep 72
Global disasters 144–145, 148–149
Global anxiety triggers 140, 148–149
Grief 126–127
Going to the gym 102
Going shopping 96

H

Having your photo taken 54–55
Heading to college/university 122–123

Helping others 150–151
How to use this book 8–9

I

Illness anxiety disorder 22
Intimacy anxiety 106–107

L

Leadership anxiety 116

M

Making friends 86–87
Mantras 37
Meditation 40–41
Meditation for sleep 70–71
Meeting new people 84–85
Menstrual cycle 64–65
Mindfulness 38–39
Moving home 124

O

Obsessive compulsive disorder 25
Online dating 103–105

P

Panic attacks 24
Perfectionism 31
Phobias 28–29
Political anxiety 141–142, 148–149
Post-traumatic stress disorder 26

Professional support 45
Public speaking 90–91

R

Redundancy 125
Rejection 74–79

S

Saying no 114–115
Sexual anxiety 106–107
Sleep 66–67
Social anxiety disorder 21
Social media 94–95
Speaking on the phone 92–93
Starting conversations 88–89
Stress of modern living 30
Study anxiety 132

T

Taking exams 134–135
3-3-3 technique 44

V

Validation 80–81
Visiting the doctor 63
Visualization 42–43

W

Workplace anxiety 128–130
Worry 14

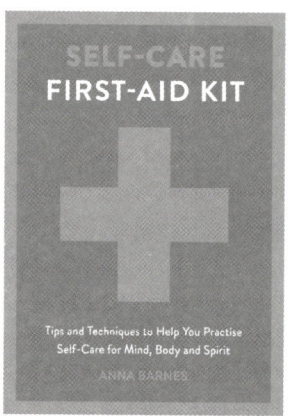

SELF-CARE FIRST-AID KIT

Tips and Techniques to Help You Practise Self-Care for Mind, Body and Spirit

Anna Barnes

ISBN: 978-1-83799-751-0 (Hardback)

This compact go-to guide is here to provide you with inspiration and advice on practising self-care for mind, body and spirit

Whether you want to explore the benefits of a digital detox or find meditation exercises to bring you instant calm, this book is here to help. The tips and techniques inside will allow you to find relief and respite when you're in urgent need of a self-care boost – simply dip into this soothing little guide to treat yourself as and when you like!

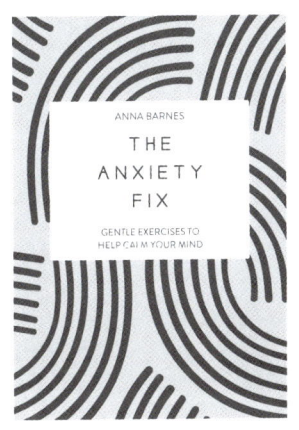

THE ANXIETY FIX

Gentle Exercises to Help Calm Your Mind

Anna Barnes

ISBN: 978-1-83799-160-0 (Paperback)

Quieten your mind with this guided journal, filled with practical tips and simple strategies for managing feelings of anxiety

Anxiety can feel like a huge obstacle to living the life you want – but it doesn't have to be! The prompts and exercises in this guided journal will help you work through your worries, develop your self-belief, learn coping strategies and more, giving you the tools to conquer your anxiety, boost your well-being and live a happier life.

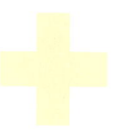

Have you enjoyed this book?
If so, why not write a review on your favourite website?

If you're interested in finding out more about our books, find us on Facebook at Summersdale Publishers, on Twitter/X at @Summersdale and on Instagram, TikTok and Bluesky at @summersdalebooks and get in touch. We'd love to hear from you!

Thanks very much for buying
this Summersdale book.

www.summersdale.com